Prescribing in Pregnancy

Prescribing in Pregnancy

Fourth edition

Edited by

Peter Rubin
Nottingham University Hospitals
Queen's Medical Centre Campus
Nottingham, UK

Margaret Ramsay
Nottingham University Hospitals
Queen's Medical Centre Campus
Nottingham, UK

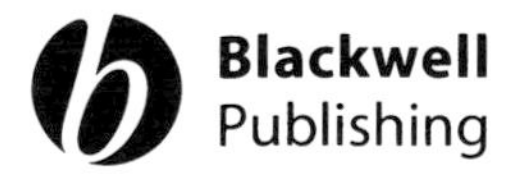

BMJ | Books

BMJ Books is an imprint of the BMJ Publishing Group Limited, used under licence

Blackwell Publishing, Inc., 350 Main Street, Malden, Massachusetts 02148-5020, USA
Blackwell Publishing Ltd, 9600 Garsington Road, Oxford OX4 2DQ, UK
Blackwell Publishing Asia Pty Ltd, 550 Swanston Street, Carlton, Victoria 3053, Australia

First published 1987
Second Edition 1995
Third Edition 2000
Fourth Edition 2008

1 2008

Library of Congress Cataloging-in-Publication Data
Prescribing in pregnancy / edited by Peter Rubin, Margaret Ramsay. – 4th ed.
p. ; cm.
ISBN 978-1-4051-4712-5 (pbk.)
1. Obstetrical pharmacology. I. Rubin, Peter C. II. Ramsay, M. M., M.D.
[DNLM: 1. Drug Therapy. 2. Pregnancy. 3. Pharmaceutical
Preparations–administration & dosage. 4. Pregnancy Complications–drug therapy.
WQ 200 P932 2007]
RG528.P74 2007
618.2'061–dc22

2007017554

ISBN: 978-1-4051-4712-5

A catalogue record for this title is available from the British Library

Set in 9.5/12pt Meridien by Aptara Inc., New Delhi, India
Printed and bound in Singapore by Markono Print Media Pte Ltd

Commissioning Editor: Mary Banks
Editorial Assistant: Victoria Pittman
Development Editor: Simone Dudziak
Production Controller: Rachel Edwards

For further information on Blackwell Publishing, visit our website:
http://www.blackwellpublishing.com

The publisher's policy is to use permanent paper from mills that operate a sustainable forestry policy, and which has been manufactured from pulp processed using acid-free and elementary chlorine-free practices. Furthermore, the publisher ensures that the text paper and cover board used have met acceptable environmental accreditation standards.

Blackwell Publishing makes no representation, express or implied, that the drug dosages in this book are correct. Readers must therefore always check that any product mentioned in this publication is used in accordance with the prescribing information prepared by the manufacturers. The author and the publishers do not accept responsibility or legal liability for any errors in the text or for the misuse or misapplication of material in this book.

Contents

Contributors

Anthony J. Avery, DM, FRCGP
Professor of Primary Health Care
Division of Primary Care
School of Community Health Sciences
Nottingham University Hospitals
Queen's Medical Centre Campus
Nottingham, UK

Anita Banerjee, BSc, MBBS, MRCP
SpR Endocrinology and Diabetes Mellitus
Endocrinology Department
Hammersmith Hospital
London, UK

Susan L. Brent, BSc (Hons), MRPharmS
Director of Pharmacy
Regional Drug and Therapeutics Centre
Wolfson Unit
Newcastle upon Tyne, UK

Mary Gayed, MBChB
Academic Foundation Year Two Doctor
City Hospital
Sandwell and West Birmingham Hospitals NHS Trust
Birmingham, UK

Anastasios Gazis, DM, MRCP
Consultant Physician
Department of Endocrinology and Diabetes
Nottingham University Hospitals
Queen's Medical Centre Campus
Nottingham, UK

Caroline Gordon, MRCP
Reader and Consultant in Rheumatology
Department of Rheumatology
Division of Immunity and Infection
Medical School
University of Birmingham
Birmingham, UK

Christine P. Hayes, MPhil, BSc (Hons)
Epilepsy Specialist Nurse
Neurosciences
Nottingham University Hospitals
Queen's Medical Centre Campus
Nottingham, UK

Mary Hepburn, BSc, MD, MRCGP, FRCOG
Consultant Obstetrician
Princess Royal Maternity
Glasgow, UK

Pauline A. Hurley, FRCOG
Consultant Obstetrics, Fetal Medicine
The Women's Centre
John Radcliffe Hospital
Oxford, UK

Conor Jamieson, BSc, PhD, MRPharmS
Principal Pharmacist – Anti-infectives
Heart of England NHS Foundation Trust
Birmingham, UK

Asma Khalil, MB, BCh
Senior Research Fellow
Homerton University Hospital
London, UK

Lena Macara, MD, FRCOG
Consultant Obstetrician
The Queen Mother's Hospital
Glasgow, UK

Kate Morel
Diabetes Nurse Specialist Manager
Brighton and Sussex University Hospitals NHS Turst
Brighton, UK

Bethan Myers, MA, MRCP, FRCPath, DTM & H
Consultant Haematologist
Department of Haematology
Nottingham University Hospitals
Queen's Medical Centre Campus
Nottingham, UK

Pat O'Brien, MRCOG
Obstetric Lead
University College London Hospitals
London, UK

Michael F. O'Donoghue, BSc, MB BS, MD, MRCP (UK)
Consultant Neurologist
Nottingham University Hospitals
Queen's Medical Centre Campus
Nottingham, UK

Margaret M. Ramsay, MA, MD, MRCP, FRCOG
Consultant in Fetomaternal Medicine
Nottingham University Hospitals
Queen's Medical Centre Campus
Nottingham, UK

Peter C. Rubin, MA, DM, FRCP
Professor of Therapeutics
Nottingham University Hospitals
Queen's Medical Centre Campus
Nottingham, UK

Jane M. Rutherford, DM, MRCOG
Consultant in Fetomaternal Medicine
Department of Obstetrics
Nottingham University Hospitals
Queen's Medical Centre Campus
Nottingham, UK

Neelam Sisodia, MBBS, MA, MRCPsych
Consultant in Perinatal Psychiatry
Perinatal Psychiatric Service
Mother and Baby Unit
Nottingham University Hospitals
Queen's Medical Centre Campus
Nottingham, UK

N.J.A. Vaughan MA, MD, FRCP
Consultant Endocrinologist
Brighton and Sussex University Hospitals Trust
Royal Sussex County Hospital
Brighton, UK

Louise Walker, RD
Specialist Diabetes Dietician
Diabetes Centre
Brighton and Sussex University Hospitals
Royal Sussex County Hospital
Brighton, UK

Tim Weller, MBChB, MD, FRCPath *(deceased)*
Previously Consultant Microbiologist
Department of Microbiology
City Hospital
Birmingham, UK

Catherine Williamson, MD, MRCP
Senior Lecturer in Obstetric Medicine
Hammersmith Hospital
Imperial College
London, UK

Preface

The use of drugs in women who are pregnant or breast feeding is a question of fine balance. Harm may befall a baby because a drug has been used, but mother and baby could suffer if a disease goes untreated. Information about the safe and effective use of drugs in pregnancy has not kept pace with the advances in other areas of therapeutics. Systematic research involving drugs in pregnancy is fraught with ethical, legal, emotional and practical difficulties and in many cases our knowledge is based on anecdote or small studies.

The purpose of this book is to bring together what is known about prescribing in pregnancy and to put that information in a clinical context. The first three editions were well received and this has encouraged us to produce a fourth edition. All chapters have been extensively revised or rewritten, with several new authors bringing their clinical experience of this challenging subject.

We would like to thank Louise Sabli who once again has done much behind-the-scenes work in contacting authors.

Acknowledgement

Dr Weller died suddenly while training for the London Marathon shortly after submitting his chapter. He had also contributed to the third edition and we gratefully acknowledge the professional manner in which he approached these tasks.

Peter Rubin
Margaret Ramsay
Nottingham

CHAPTER 1

Identifying fetal abnormalities

Lena M. Macara

Key points

- Days 18–55 postconception is the time of maximal teratogenic potential when most organs are differentiating
- Teratogenic effects of medications may affect both organ structure and organ function
- Detailed ultrasound assessment of the fetus by trained personnel should detect most major structural abnormalities, but minor abnormalities are often undetected
- Patients at risk of neural tube defects (NTDs) should have 5 mg of folic acid daily for a minimum of 6 wk prior to conception

Introduction

It is estimated that 2–3% of all pregnancies in the United Kingdom are affected by congenital abnormality. Almost half of these abnormalities remain of uncertain aetiology, a further 25% may be linked to a variety of genetic problems and only 2% are likely to be associated with environmental factors that include medicinal products.

While this is a very small proportion of all birth defects, it is a critical group, since the avoidance of some medications will prevent these abnormalities from occurring. For parents and physicians, it is therefore one of the few areas in which the outcome of pregnancy can be influenced.

Prescribing in Pregnancy, 4th edition. Edited by Peter Rubin and Margaret Ramsay,
 ISBN: 978-1-4051-4712-5.

Both the number and spectrum of medicinal products available, 'over the counter' and on a prescribed basis, has expanded enormously in the last decade. At any given time, over 80% of women in childbearing years are using some type of medication and around 50% of pregnant women are prescribed a medication other than a vitamin or supplement during pregnancy [1,2].

This chapter aims to guide clinicians on normal pregnancy development, the options currently available to assess fetal development in utero and the spectrum of abnormalities linked with drug use during pregnancy, which may be detected prior to delivery. The following chapters will provide guidance on prescribing in pregnancy, highlighting those drugs that should be avoided in pregnancy and offering direction on those medications with least risk to the pregnancy while ensuring that the underlying medical issues are dealt with.

Embryonic and fetal development

It is clear from practice that not all drugs affect a pregnancy in an identical manner or to equal degrees of severity. This is due to the rapid but staggered sequence of events that occur as two cells quickly multiply to form the embryo and fetus we recognise. Understanding the order and timing of this process may help us to understand which organ systems are likely to be affected at each stage of pregnancy and anticipate the possible long-term effects which may ensue.

Fetal development can be divided into three main stages: the pre-differentiation or pre-embryonic phase; from conception until 17 days postconception, just after the first missed period; the embryonic stage from 3 to 8 weeks postconception and the fetal phase from week 8 until term.

During the pre-differentiation stage, the cells of the conceptus divide rapidly and remain totipotential. Any insult to the pregnancy during this phase seems to have an 'all or nothing' effect. If most of the cells are affected, the pregnancy is spontaneously miscarried but when only some cells are affected, the remaining totipotent cells appear to replace the damaged cells without any apparent long-term deleterious effect. Most women will not yet have missed their first period and therefore may not realise that they are pregnant.

During the embryonic period, these cells differentiate and form definitive organ systems (Figure 1.1). Since the cells have now

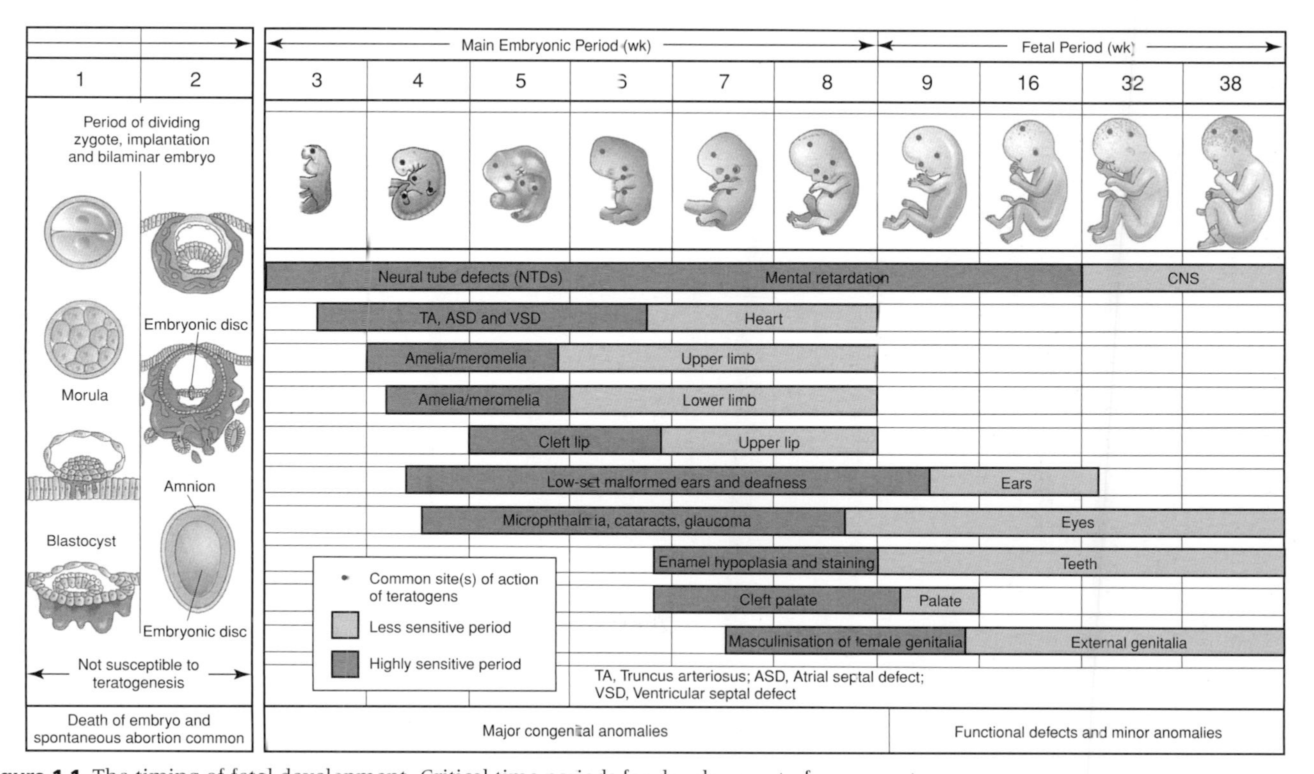

Figure 1.1 The timing of fetal development. Critical time periods for development of organ systems.
Reprinted from Figure 8.15 from Moore et al: The Developing Human: Clinically Oriented Embryology, 6/E ©1998 with permission from Elsevier

differentiated, if they are extensively damaged, permanent effects are likely to occur in the end organ. Although the embryonic period is short, each end organ has a window of maximal susceptibility when the teratogenic insults are likely to be most severe. In some circumstances, the effects may be dosage dependent.

The fetal period is primarily a time of growth and maturation, and most drugs are therefore unlikely to cause significant structural defects. However, organs such as the cerebral cortex, the gastrointestinal tract and the renal glomeruli continue to differentiate and develop throughout pregnancy and into the neonatal period. These organs therefore remain vulnerable to growth or functional damage by medicinal products during the later stages of pregnancy. These are often more subtle changes and frequently will only become evident as the neonate grows and develops. The teratogenic effect of a drug administered during pregnancy may therefore be easily overlooked.

Since the nature and degree of teratogenic effects on a pregnancy is largely determined by the stage of development at which exposure occurs, the gestational age of the pregnancy at presentation must first be determined. Thereafter, careful documentation of the nature, dosage and duration of the products used should be recorded for future reference.

Determining gestational age in pregnancy

The pregnancy hormone human chorionic gonadotrophin can be detected in urine around the time of the first missed period, and in serum even earlier. Transvaginal ultrasound (TV) can now visualise a pregnancy 2–3 weeks following conception, though viability of the pregnancy can only be determined once a fetal heartbeat is seen 3–4 weeks postconception by TV scan or 4 weeks postconception with an abdominal ultrasound scan. Thereafter, standard measurements of the total fetal length, fetal femur length and fetal skull diameter may be obtained to calculate the gestational age of the fetus. Pregnancy is divided into three trimesters: the first trimester from the time of the last menstrual period, week 0 until week 12, the second trimester from week 12 until week 24 and the third trimester from week 24 until term.

Evaluating fetal anatomy

With good quality ultrasound machinery, basic fetal anatomy, confirming integrity of the skull bones, the abdominal wall, upper

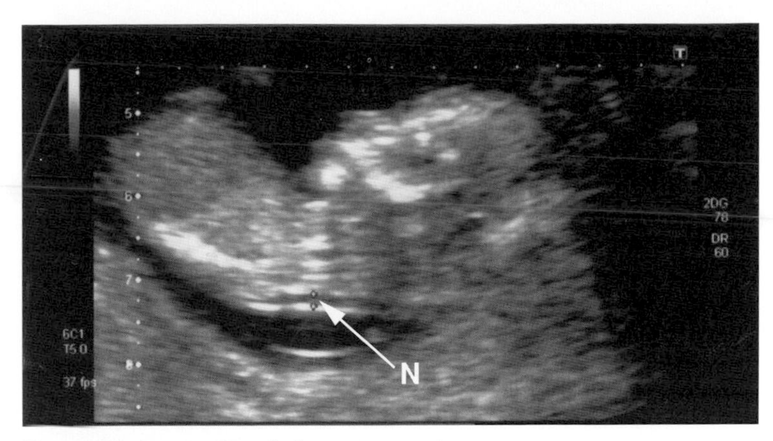

Figure 1.2 A normal nuchal measurement.

and lower limbs, and a fetal stomach, may now be identified by the 12th week of gestation. Many units also assess the depth of nuchal fluid present at the fetal neck (Figure 1.2). This, in combination with biochemical parameters, can quantify the risk of chromosomal abnormality. In addition, a large nuchal measurement (Figure 1.3) is associated with increased risk of fetal cardiac abnormality, and detailed assessment of the heart at a later gestation is advised. A more extensive examination of fetal anatomy in the first trimester is performed in selected units. At 11–12 weeks,

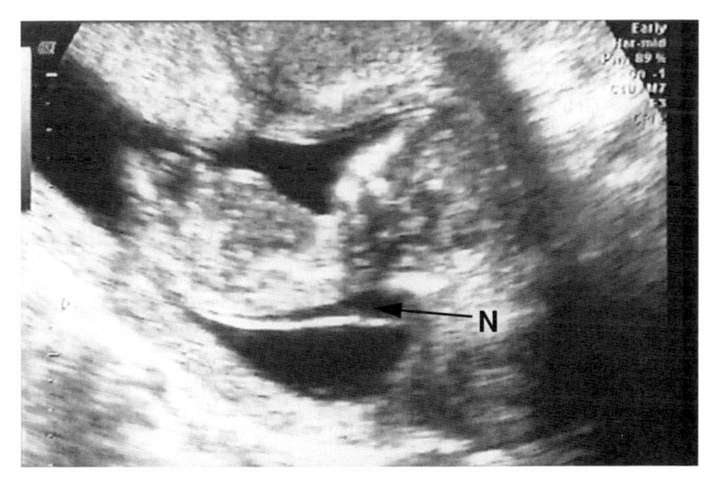

Figure 1.3 Increased nuchal measurement.

a complete examination of the fetus can be achieved in only 50–60% of cases. With the addition of TV examination, and deferring the examination until 12–14 completed weeks of pregnancy, 90% of pregnancies can be successfully examined [3,4]. While this option offers early reassurance to parents, most departments do not have the trained personnel, nor the resources to offer this level of detailed ultrasound examination in the first trimester.

For the majority of patients, fetal anatomy is still evaluated between 18 and 20 weeks of gestation – 'the routine anomaly scan'. Though this is recommended for all pregnancies, at the time of writing, routine anomaly scans are still not available within some major health board areas in Scotland and England unless specific indications such as medication in pregnancy are highlighted.

Many groups have evaluated second trimester ultrasound examination and confirmed that 70–90% of significant abnormalities should be detected [5,6]. There are several reasons for this variation. The list of structures that are deemed essential to examine in each pregnancy is at the discretion of individual units, and many departments do not examine the fetal heart, face or limbs in detail. Therefore an examination may be complete as per department protocol but may not evaluate the very organ most likely to be affected by specific drugs. In addition, some anomalies such as congenital diaphragmatic hernia, microcephaly and hydrocephalus may not be evident until the late second trimester, after the time of a standard detailed scan, and other functional problems of organs like the brain or kidney will remain unidentified until the neonatal period. Moreover dysmorphic features, such as flatting of facial bones or other soft markers, will not be seen on standard ultrasound scans.

In view of these facts, women who are at risk of congenital abnormality as a result of medication during pregnancy must be highlighted at every stage of referral to ensure that a full detailed ultrasound examination is performed, and at times repeated, at an appropriate stage of pregnancy.

Within the last couple of years, 3D ultrasound technology has enabled more detailed examination of the fetal surface and proved particularly useful in assessment of the fetal face (Figure 1.4). Three-dimensional images often prove very difficult both to obtain and to interpret at less than 24 weeks of gestation. Where exclusion or confirmation of fetal problems such as cleft lip is required, referral to a tertiary centre with 3D ultrasound experience may be indicated.

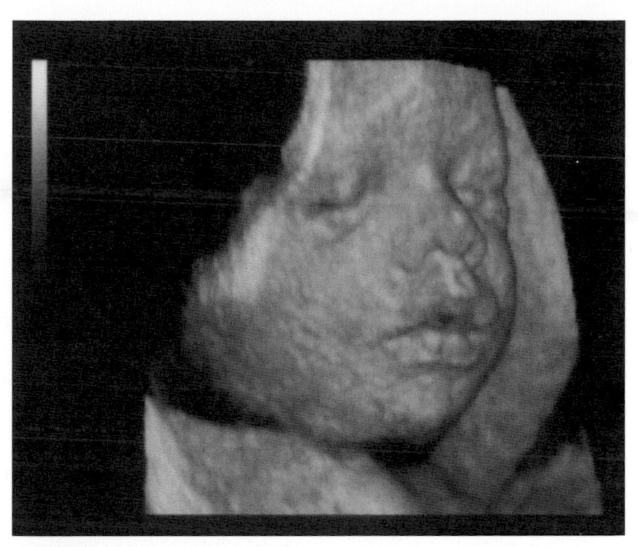

Figure 1.4 Three-dimensional ultrasound image of a normal fetal face (24 weeks of gestation).

Once a fetal abnormality has been identified on ultrasound, further information may be obtained from fetal MRI studies. To date, these studies are primarily a research tool, evaluating, for example, if MRI can predict the severity of spina bifida or the degree of fetal lung development in congenital diaphragmatic hernia.

Pregnancy management

Pre-pregnancy: reducing the risk of fetal abnormality

Ideally all pregnancy management should commence in the preconception period. Clinicians need to be aware of the potential effects of the more commonly prescribed medications as outlined in Table 1.1. Where possible, non essential drugs should be stopped and polypharmacy reduced to a monotherapy, selecting those with the least teratogenic profile. Women on antihypertensive and anticonvulsant therapy, on treatment for long-standing rheumatoid problems and on anticoagulants and immunosuppressants should meet with their clinician to optimise drug therapy prior to conception. As evident from Figure 1.1, much of critical organ development will occur before most women attend for a booking appointment, and therefore stopping any drug abruptly at week 10–12 is of little value to either the woman or her fetus. *The risk of*

Table 1.1 Medications associated with specific congenital abnormalities

Fetal effects	Medication
Central nervous system	
Neural tube defects (spina bifida, anencephaly, encephalocele)	Sodium valproate, hydantoin, rifampicin
Other structural defects	Retinoids, warfarin, carbamazepine, sodium valproate
Mental impairment	Anti-epileptics, alcohol
Cardiac	Lithium, thalidomide, retinoids, paroxetine valproate
Renal	
Oliguria, renal failure	NSAIDS, ACE inhibitors, COX-2 inhibitors
Gastrointestinal tract	
Necrotising enterocolitis	Augmentin, NSAIDS
Gastoschisis	Cannabis, recreational drugs
Facial	
Cleft lip and palate	Rifampicin, retinoids, steroids Sodium talproate, benzodiazepines
Abnormal facial features	Alcohol
Skeletal	Thalidomide, cocaine, tetracyclines
Growth restriction	β-blockers, alcohol, valproate, amphetamines
Placental abruption	Aspirin, warfarin, crack cocaine

NTDs in pregnancy can be reduced by the use of high-dose folic acid. In order to be effective, 5 mg of folic acid must be taken for at least 6 weeks prior to conception and continued until the 12th week of pregnancy. Any woman of childbearing age who is on medication associated with a risk of NTD should be prescribed this higher dose of folic acid [7,8]. Folic acid may also reduce the risks of facial clefting in patients on anticonvulsant therapy, but this is based on less clear data [9].

Antenatal care: assessing fetal development

Once pregnancy is confirmed, the patient should be referred to an obstetric unit for antenatal care. Having confirmed gestational age and basic fetal anatomy, a full detailed ultrasound scan should be arranged in the second trimester. The presence of an increased nuchal measurement should stimulate a detailed examination in the second trimester, with particular attention to the fetal heart.

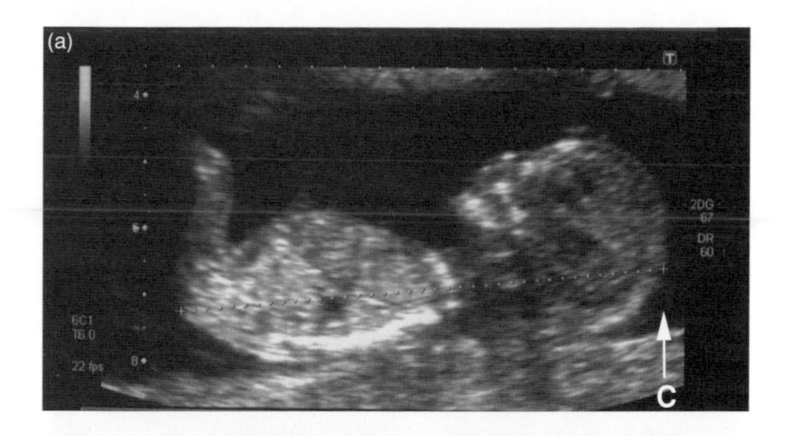

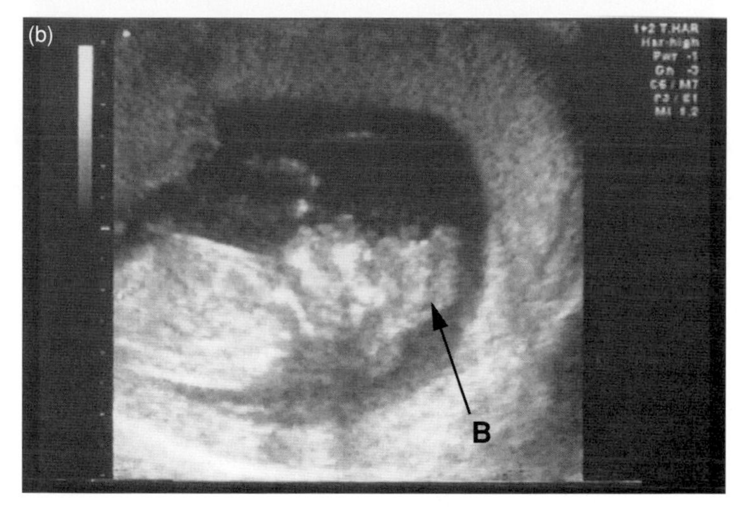

Figure 1.5 (a) A normal mid-sagittal image of a 12-week fetus with normal cranial bones (C) visible; (b) a 12-week fetus with anencephaly. The cranial vault is absent and fetal brain tissue (B) seen to float freely.

Antenatal care: common fetal abnormalities detected by ultrasound

Central nervous system

Failure of the neural tube to close may result in a range of defects. Anencephaly, failure of the skull bones to develop, is incompatible with independent life and should be detected in all pregnancies by 12 weeks of gestation, if the skull bones are not clearly visualised on ultrasound (Figures 1.5a–1.5b). Although spina bifida

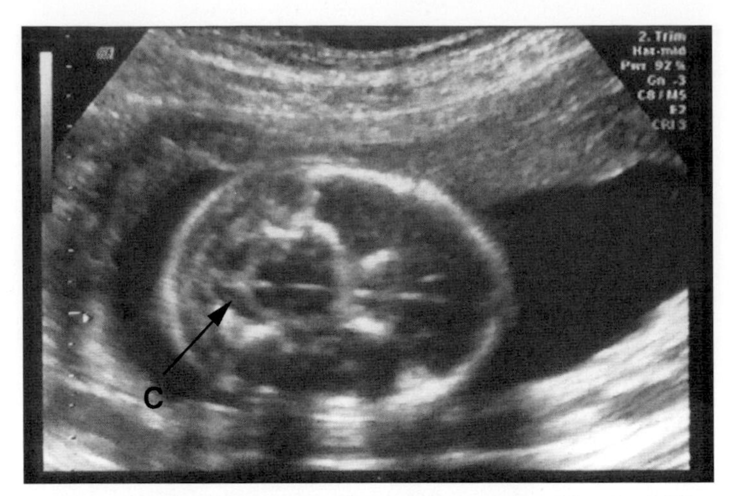

Figure 1.6 Arnold–Chiari-type malformation in a baby with spina bifida, showing the abnormal cerebellum (C).

usually affects the lower vertebrae, up to 80% of babies will also have intracranial signs in the second trimester, due to an abnormal cerebellum and hydrocephalus (Figure 1.6). With current ultrasound imaging, amniocentesis, to detect the acetyl cholinesterase band specific for NTD, should no longer be required. Over 90% of NTDs should be detected with second trimester ultrasound assessment. Other abnormalities such as Dandy–Walker-type malformations (Figure 1.7) and cerebral cysts should be detected antenatally.

Cardiovascular system

Even in specialist units where the heart and outflow tracts are examined, 70–80% of abnormalities are identified antenatally, but detection rates as low as 15% have been reported in more general population studies [10,11]. When a normal four-chamber view of the heart is seen (Figure 1.8), 40% of anomalies should be excluded.

Facial clefting

The fetal position, the small size of the alveolar ridge, fetal limbs placed in front of the face and the increasing maternal body mass index in the population can make this a technically difficult area

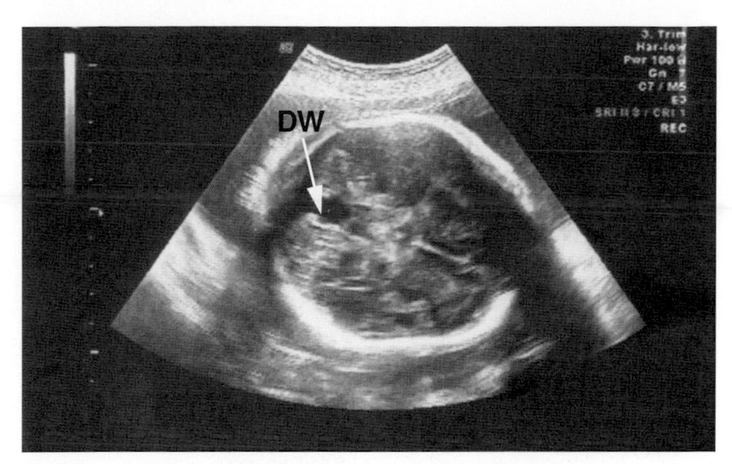

Figure 1.7 Ultrasound of a fetal head. A large echolucent area (Dandy–Walker (DW)-type malformation) is present in the posterior fossa.

to examine completely. When complete views of the face are obtained, 50–70% of cleft lip with or without cleft palate is recognised (Figures 1.9a–1.9b). Isolated cleft palates have *not* been detected prenatally, most probably because the fetal tongue, of the same echogenicity as the palate, occludes the defect.

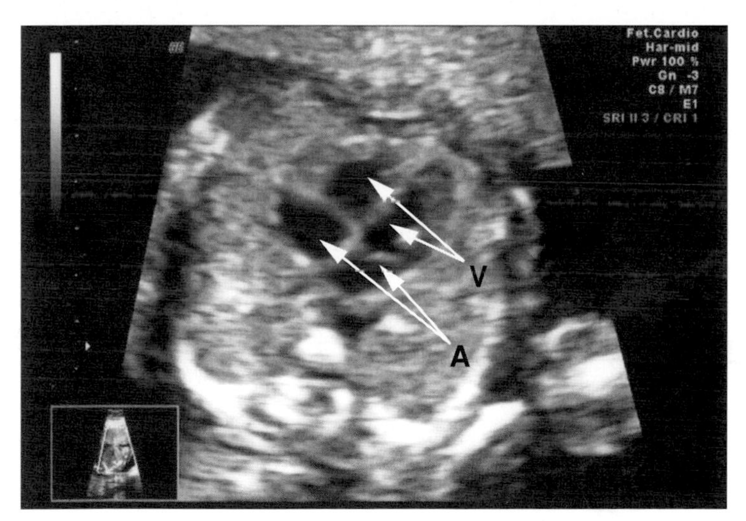

Figure 1.8 A normal four-chamber view of the heart showing the ventricles (V) and atria (A).

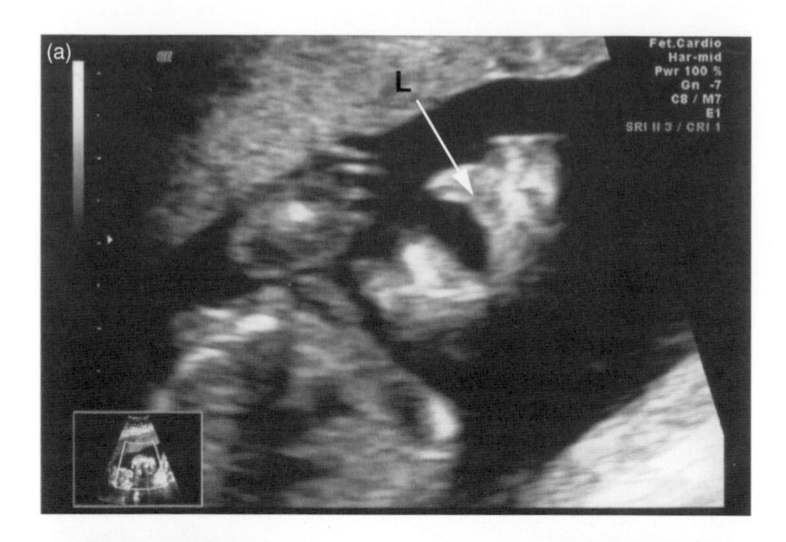

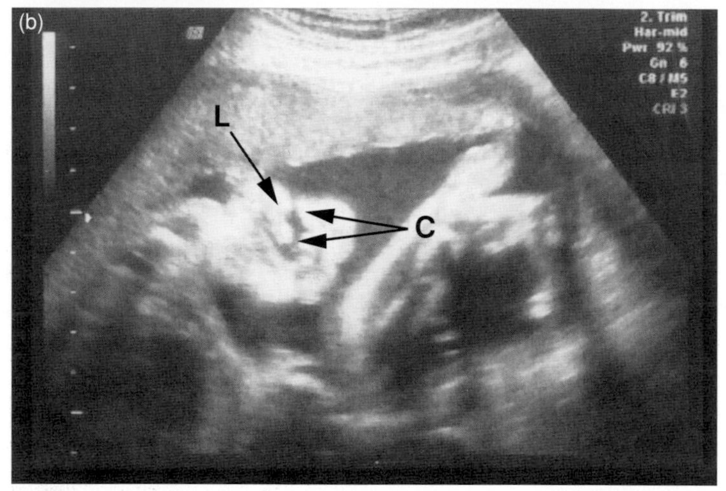

Figure 1.9 (a) Normal profile of fetal lips (L) in the second trimester; (b) profile of fetal lips showing the upper lips (L) with a large cleft (C) present.

Other craniofacial abnormalities such as hypertelorism or a thin upper lip cannot be identified with current 2D scan imaging. With increasing experience of 3D imaging, these 'minor' soft markers may well be visualised, but the value of obtaining this information, particularly in the third trimester may be questionable.

Skeletal problems

It is relatively easy to measure fetal limbs during pregnancy, but many subtle deviations in growth do not present until the third trimester, well beyond the time of detailed anomaly scanning. Since assessment of fetal limb length is routine in most departments, gross defects of the type associated with thalidomide should easily be detected by 18 weeks. Where teratogenesis is suspected, careful inspection of the hands, feet and digits should be made. Other aetiologies for skeletal problems, such as chromosome problems, are common and should be excluded before attributing any defects to drug ingestion.

Fetal abnormality: parental options

Once an abnormality is identified, parents should be counselled regarding the nature of the abnormality and any associated problems. Where indicated, parents should be offered a diagnostic test to confirm the fetal karyotype. When the abnormality is likely to have significant risk of physical or mental handicap, parents have the option to terminate the pregnancy. Beyond 22 weeks completed gestation, the fetal heart must be stopped prior to delivery, and hence every effort should be made to facilitate early diagnosis whenever possible. When parents opt to continue with the pregnancy, management of the pregnancy, labour and delivery may need to be modified and depending on the facilities available, parents may need to be referred to regional centres.

Antenatal care: ongoing care

Women on medication associated with growth restriction, poor placental function, impaired renal function or premature closure of the ductus arteriosus require ongoing monitoring during the pregnancy, and appropriate ultrasound assessment in the third trimester should be arranged.

Summary and key points

Most congenital abnormalities are not related to drug use in pregnancy. Where drugs are known to be associated with structural abnormalities, a detailed ultrasound scan in the second trimester should be offered to confirm normal fetal development. When an abnormality is detected, parents have the option of termination of the pregnancy where the problem is substantial or that of planned delivery when early paediatric input is beneficial. Detailed ultrasound scans cannot detect functional abnormalities such as mental retardation or minor problems such as dysmorphic features. In the event of this being detected at birth, other common causes of mental retardation must be excluded before a specific drug is blamed. It is prudent for all clinicians presented with a woman who has used medication during pregnancy to ensure careful documentation at the time of presentation, as many functional problems are often not identified until the child is several months old and recollecting the timing of drug exposure and the investigations performed can be difficult at a later date.

References

1 Kaufman DW, Kelly JP, Rosenberg L, et al. Recent patterns of medication use in the ambulatory adult population of the United States: the Slone survey. *JAMA* 2002;**287**(3):337–44.
2 Andrade SE, Gurwitz JH, Davis RL, et al. Prescription drug use in pregnancy. *Am J Obstet Gynaecol* 2004;**191**(2):398–407.
3 Economides DL, Whitlow BJ, Braithwaite JM. Ultrasonography in the detection of fetal abnormalities in early pregnancy. *BJOG* 1999;**106**: 516.
4 Souka AP, Pilalis A, Kavalakis Y, Komas Y, Antsaklis P, Anstakalis A. Assessment of fetal anatomy at the 11–14 week examination. *Ultrasound Obstet Gynaecol* 2004;**24**:730–4.
5 Chitty LS, Hunt GH, Moore J, Lobb MO. Effectiveness of routine ultrasonography in detecting fetal structural problems in a low risk population. *BMJ* 1991;**303**:1165–9.
6 Smith NC, Hau C. A six year study of the antenatal detection of fetal abnormality in six Scottish health boards. *Br J Obstet Gynaecol* 1999;**106**:206–12.
7 Reynolds EH. Anti-convulsants, folic acid and epilepsy. *Lancet* 1973; **1**:1376–88.
8 MRC Vitamin Research Study Group. Prevention of neural tube defects: results of the MRC vitamin study. *Lancet* 1991;**338**:131–9.
9 Shaw GM, Lammer EJ, Wasserman CR, O'Malley CD, Tolarova MM. Risks of oro-facial clefts in children born to women using multivitamins containing folic acid periconceprtionally. *Lancet* 1995;**346**: 399.

10 Allan LD. Echocardiographic detection of congenital heart disease in the fetus: present and future. *Br Heart J* 1995;**74**:103–6.
11 Westin M, Saltvedt S, Bergman G, et al. Routine ultrasound examination at 12 or 18 gestational weeks for prenatal detection of major congenital heart malformations? A randomised controlled trial comparing 36,299 fetuses. *Br J Obstet Gynaecol* 2006;**113**:675–82.

CHAPTER 2
Treatment of common, minor and self-limiting conditions

Anthony J. Avery, Susan L. Brent

This chapter deals with the management of some common, minor and self-limiting conditions that may occur during pregnancy. Since most of these are minor, we would emphasise the importance of non-drug treatments and manoeuvres such as intermittent drug use to limit exposure of the fetus to any medication that may be used. Exposure of the fetus during the first 10 weeks of gestation is when there is greatest risk of congenital defect, since this is the period of organogenesis. However, drugs taken during the later stages of pregnancy may give rise to more subtle deformities. In addition, neonates can experience withdrawal symptoms associated with certain drugs prescribed during pregnancy. Despite these problems, there is still a need to use drugs to relieve troublesome symptoms in some cases.

Key points

1 Where possible, try non-drug treatments first
2 In selecting drugs:
- choose the one that has the best safety record over time
- avoid newer drugs, unless safety has been clearly established
- do not assume that over-the-counter drugs and herbal medicines are safe

Prescribing in Pregnancy, 4th edition. Edited by Peter Rubin and Margaret Ramsay,
 ISBN: 978-1-4051-4712-5.

– for manufacturers' advice on cautions and contraindications in pregnancy, check the latest version of the summary of product characteristics

3 In deciding on doses and treatment courses:
– avoid the first 10 wk of gestation if possible
– use the lowest effective dose
– use the drug for the shortest period of time necessary
– where possible, use drugs intermittently rather than continuously
– if chronic use is indicated, consider withdrawing or reducing the dose of the agent before the expected date of delivery, taking into consideration the potential risks and benefits of such a strategy

In this chapter we focus on drugs in pregnancy for the following:

- Symptoms affecting the gastrointestinal tract
- Minor ailments involving the respiratory tract
- Pain
- Common fungal infections
- Common infestations

A summary of the drugs discussed under each of above is given in Table 2.1. We conclude the chapter by giving advice on inadvertent drug use in pregnancy.

The gastrointestinal tract

Nausea and vomiting

A substantial proportion of women suffer from nausea, vomiting, or both during the early stages of pregnancy, typically between 6 and 12 weeks of gestation. Although known colloquially as 'morning sickness', the symptoms can occur at any time of the day. The cause is poorly understood, although thought to be related to raised levels of human chorionic gonadotrophin. Higher blood levels of this hormone are seen in multiple pregnancy and this is thought to explain the more severe symptoms sometimes experienced. Most women who suffer symptoms of nausea and vomiting manage to limit these by avoiding foods likely to exacerbate symptoms and by eating at times of the day when symptoms are less severe. Simple advice such as eating smaller meals that are high in carbohydrate

Table 2.1 Drugs used for common, minor and self-limiting conditions and their safety in pregnancy

Drug	Trimester 1	Trimester 2	Trimester 3	Comment
		Nausea and vomiting		
Cyclizine	1	1	1	Widest experience with promethazine and cyclizine
Promethazine	1	1	1	
Metoclopramide	1	1	1	
Domperidone	1	1	1	
Prochlorperazine	1	1	1	
Hyoscine hydrobromide	2	2	2	
		Symptoms affecting the gastrointestinal tract		
Antacids	1	1	1	
Alginate antacids, e.g., Gaviscon, Algicon	1	1	1	
Cimetidine	1	1	1	
Ranitidine	1	1	1	
Omeprazole	1	1	1	
Lansoprazole	2	2	2	
Lactulose	1	1	1	
Senna	1	1	2	
Bisacodyl	1	1	1	
Docusate	2	2	2	
Glycerin suppositories	1	1	1	
Loperamide	2	2	2	
Co-phenotrope	2	2	2	
		Minor ailments involving the respiratory tract		
Topical sympathomimetics, e.g., xylometazoline	1	1	1	
Intranasal corticosteroids	1	1	1	
Antitussives				
Dextromethorphan	2	2	2	
Pholcodine	2	2	2	
Sodium cromoglicate drops	1	1	1	
Beclometasone nasal spray	1	1	1	
Chlorphenamine	1	1	1	
Promethazine	1	1	1	

(*Continued*)

Table 2.1 (*Continued*)

Drug	Trimester 1	Trimester 2	Trimester 3	Comment
Cetirizine	2	2	2	
Loratadine	2	2	2	
Fexofenadine	3	3	3	
Levocetirizine	3	3	3	
Desloratadine	3	3	3	
		Pain		
Paracetamol	1	1	1	
Aspirin (at analgesic doses)	2	2	3	See text for comments on low-dose aspirin
NSAIDs	2	1	3	Ibuprofen preferred
COX 2s	3	3	3	
Opioids including codeine, morphine, pethidine, fentanyl, hydromorphone, oxycodone	1	1	2	Newborn infant may be opioid dependent
Tramadol	2	2	2	
Sumatriptan	3	3	3	
Ergotamine	3	3	3	
		Common fungal infections		
Clotrimazole (topical)	1	1	1	Nystatin less effective than clotrimazole
Nystatin (topical)	1	1	1	
Fluconazole	2	2	2	Avoid high dose/regular use
Ketoconazole	3	3	3	
Itraconazole	3	3	3	
Griseofulvin	3	3	3	
Terbinafine	3	3	3	
		Common infestations		
Malathion	1	1	1	
Permethrin	1	1	1	Aqueous preparations preferable
Phenothrin	1	1	1	
Carbaryl	2	2	2	
Piperazine	2	1	1	
Mebendazole	2	1	1	

Refer to text before using this table. Use any drug in lowest possible dose for shortest time.

1, drug probably safe during pregnancy; 2, safety uncertain, or insufficient data; 3, unsafe, or very limited experience.

and low in fat and avoidance of large volumes of fluid (substituting smaller volumes more frequently) may be helpful. It is also important to maintain adequate hydration, especially in hyperemesis.

More severe vomiting may occur in a minority of women and can lead to dehydration, ketosis and weight loss, requiring admission to hospital. If nausea and vomiting are severe, drug treatment may be justified. Controlled trials have not been done and there is little evidence of comparative efficacy of drugs in relieving symptoms. There are, however, data available for outcomes following the use of some antiemetic drugs. One meta-analysis of 24 studies involving over 200,000 women exposed mainly to antihistamines concluded that there was no increased risk of teratogenicity associated with the use of such drugs [1]. A number of other drugs have been used, including the dopamine antagonists metoclopramide and domperidone, as well as phenothiazine, prochlorperazine. These have not been associated with a teratogenic effect, although the studies have involved smaller numbers of women than with the antihistamines [2].

More recently, a Cochrane review [3] has reported on the effectiveness of different methods for treating nausea and vomiting in early pregnancy, including antihistamines, ginger, pyridoxine and acupuncture or acupressure. Of the drugs considered, pyridoxine (in doses of 10–25 mg, three times daily) was least likely to cause side effects but appears more useful in the control of nausea than vomiting. Hyoscine hydrobromide, available as a transdermal patch, has not been shown to have an increased incidence of birth defects, although the numbers of women exposed are relatively small. It should be reserved for use only where other agents with more experience of use have failed to relieve symptoms [4].

A single trial of fresh ginger root was included in the Cochrane review [3] and benefit was reported for both vomiting and nausea, with no adverse effects described. In the same review, mixed results from trials of acupressure or acupuncture were reported with no clear demonstration of increased efficacy over sham or dummy acupressure or standard dietary and lifestyle advice. We are not aware of any controlled studies of morning sickness using homeopathic remedies.

The management of hyperemesis gravidarum may involve the use of corticosteroids or the 5HT3 antagonist ondansetron, although few published data are currently available for either agent.

Gastro-oesophageal reflux and heartburn

Gastro-oesophageal reflux and heartburn are reported by a substantial proportion of women in pregnancy. The symptoms are common in pregnancy, principally because of a fall in the lower oesophageal sphincter pressure, which is probably related to rising levels of progesterone [5]. The fall in lower oesophageal sphincter pressure is evident during all three trimesters. According to one small study, it reaches its lowest point at 36 weeks of gestation and returns to normal postpartum [6]. Symptoms are similar to those that occur in the non-pregnant state. Conservative measures such as avoidance of eating late in the evening or before retiring, raising the head of the bed by 10–15 cm and avoidance of fatty or strongly spiced foods may be helpful.

Antacids containing calcium, magnesium or aluminium may be useful and are generally considered safe, but it is important to consider using 'balanced' formulations (of magnesium and aluminium) to avoid problems with diarrhoea or constipation. Preparations containing alginates are largely not absorbed and are considered safe to use. Sucralfate is a mucosal protective agent which is not absorbed in significant amounts and has been shown to be effective in relieving heartburn and regurgitation during pregnancy [7].

Histamine H_2-blocking drugs are frequently used to treat gastro-oesophageal reflux in non-pregnant patients. Data from animal studies and anecdotal reports in humans are reassuring about the use of these drugs in pregnancy, although a possible anti-androgen effect has been identified in rats given cimetidine [8]. Follow-up of 553 women exposed to H_2-blockers in one study did not demonstrate any increase in malformations compared to controls – the largest group (of 330 women) received ranitidine [9]. Given this evidence, ranitidine may be considered the H_2-blocker of choice where antacids and lifestyle changes have proved ineffective.

Proton pump inhibitors (PPIs) have become widely used in the treatment of gastro-oesophageal reflux in recent years. Animal toxicity studies have shown increased embryo and fetal mortality in rats and rabbits given doses of omeprazole far in excess of those administered to humans [10]. One prospective study of 113 women who took omeprazole during the period of organogenesis found no increased incidence of major malformations over a control group [11]. There have been, however, several reports of anencephaly [12]. Despite this, omeprazole is now one of the relatively few drugs licensed for use in pregnancy. Less information is available for lansoprazole, although it has not been shown to have teratogenic effects in animal reproductive studies [13]. A recent prospective case series of pregnancy outcomes following maternal treatment with PPIs, including lansoprazole, has been published. The incidence of malformations was in line with the overall malformation rate for high-risk pregnancies held on the centre's database [14]. The small numbers involved limit the conclusions that can be drawn from the study, and PPIs remain a third-line option.

Constipation

Constipation in pregnancy is common, with rising levels of progesterone affecting gut motility. Consumption of iron preparations and aluminium-containing antacids may also contribute to symptoms. Principles of treatment of constipation are similar to those in the non-pregnant state. First-line treatment should involve increasing the intake of fruit (dried as well as fresh) and vegetables. Fluid intake should also be increased. Bulking agents such as ispaghula husk (e.g., Fybogel®, Regulan®) taken with plenty of fluid may be helpful. Lactulose is not appreciably absorbed and may also be helpful, although there is not extensive literature to support its use. The use of the stimulant laxative bisacodyl as a third-line agent throughout pregnancy has been suggested due to its low systemic absorption [15]. Senna is not thought to be teratogenic [12], although it may stimulate uterine contractions in the third trimester [16], and it may be advisable to avoid its use close to term. Docusate sodium has not been linked to specific congenital defects and may be considered for use in low doses as a fourth-line agent. Purgatives containing magnesium or sodium salts as the principal ingredient may cause electrolyte disturbances and are best avoided. Glycerol (glycerin) suppositories are unlikely to have adverse effects on the fetus.

Diarrhoea

Diarrhoea during pregnancy has similar causes to that in the non-pregnant patients, and should be investigated according to the presenting symptoms and signs. Gastroenteritis is the most common cause of diarrhoea in the childbearing years and is usually self-limiting. Treatment should be aimed at maintaining hydration, and this may be of critical importance, given the adverse effects of dehydration on the fetus. Oral rehydration solutions should be used if necessary. Use of antidiarrhoeal drugs is best avoided as experience is limited.

Diphenoxylate with atropine (co-phenotrope: Lomotil®) has not been found to be teratogenic in animals. One report suggested problems with this combination in humans [17], but the timing of administration was not consistent with the defects found. A small study reported no malformations in seven infants exposed during the first trimester [18].

No published reports linking loperamide with congenital defects have been identified [12]. A small prospective study reported that women exposed to loperamide throughout pregnancy tended to have smaller babies, although the explanation is unclear [19]. Where short-term use is necessary, loperamide may be an option.

Haemorrhoids

Although many adults suffer with haemorrhoids, these are particularly common in pregnancy. Treatment is similar to that in the non-pregnant individuals: avoidance of constipation, treatment with bulk-forming laxatives [20] or use of a bland astringent cream if necessary.

The upper respiratory tract

Upper respiratory tract infections (URTIs) and hay fever are common problems for women of childbearing age. Below we discuss the appropriateness of using antimicrobial agents in URTI. We then comment on the safety of drugs used for symptomatic treatment of upper respiratory problems.

The role of antibiotics

In patients with symptoms of the common cold, research suggests that there is no indication for using antibiotics [21]. If sinusitis develops, most studies suggest that antibiotics reduce the duration of symptoms, and therefore their use may be justified [22]. Nevertheless, one should remember that most patients will make a full recovery from sinusitis whether they receive antibiotics or not, and this may influence treatment choices in pregnancy.

A meta-analysis of studies involving the treatment of sore throat with antimicrobial agents suggests that treatment confers only modest benefits [23]. For example, the symptoms of half of patients settle within 3 days and 14 patients need to be treated to prevent one of them having an additional day of sore throat after 1 week. There is a trend towards decreased risk of glomerulonephritis with antibiotic treatment [23]. The incidence of this complication, however, is so low in Western societies that it is difficult to justify the use of antibiotics for this reason alone.

Overall, we would suggest not prescribing antibiotics for pregnant women with URTIs unless symptoms are particularly distressing. For patients with tonsillitis, it may be worth doing a throat swab before deciding whether to treat.

Symptomatic treatments for common upper respiratory problems

Given that the treatment of URTIs is essentially symptomatic, it is important to focus on the safety of preparations available and to recognise that non-pharmacological treatments such as steam inhalation may help [24]. Over-the-counter preparations for colds contain a diversity of ingredients. Frequently the principal ingredient is paracetamol or aspirin (see section on *Pain and the use of analgesics in pregnancy* for more details of these drugs). Other ingredients may include sympathomimetics, antihistamines, non-steroidal anti-inflammatory agents and stimulants such as caffeine. Preparations with a multiplicity of ingredients are best avoided, and it is probably safest to give paracetamol alone if a drug is needed for pyrexia or malaise. Sympathomimetics may help with early symptoms of nasal congestion [25], but they have diminished effect over time and may cause rebound congestion. Nose drops or nasal sprays are preferable to systemic preparations if treatment is given. If a woman wishes to use a particular favourite cold remedy, its safety should be checked with the manufacturer; ingredients in such preparations may change from time to time without notice.

Cough

There is no good evidence for or against the use of over-the-counter medications for acute cough [26]. Weak opioids such as codeine, pholcodine or dextromethorphan are often used with the intention of suppressing cough, although codeine, in particular, appears to be no more effective than placebo [26]. Expectorants and mucolytics are generally considered ineffective, but one trial showed that adults find guaifenesin helpful and another small trial showed reduction in frequent cough with Bisolvon®, a mucolytic preparation that is not available in the UK [26]. More evidence is needed to establish the safety of many over-the-counter drugs in pregnancy [27].

Hay fever

Hay fever may be problematic for some women during pregnancy. Avoidance of the precipitating allergen, if known, can reduce the need for medication. Topical treatments should generally be tried before systemic therapy in order to reduce exposure of the fetus to drugs. Sodium cromoglicate eye drops are considered to be safe as the systemic dose is very small [28]. Topical corticosteroid preparations in nasal sprays are agents of choice for rhinitis and appear to be safe in the relatively small doses used for hay fever [29]. The use of systemic corticosteroids should be avoided if possible, and there is no indication for depot injections [30]. Topical sympathomimetics have been discussed above. The problem with using these in hay fever is that prolonged use may cause rebound nasal congestion.

If a systemic antihistamine is considered essential, older sedating agents such as chlorphenamine or promethazine are preferable to the newer non-sedating agents, on the grounds of more extensive safety data [31]. Limited experience with cetirizine has not suggested any increased risk and it may be considered a suitable second choice where sedation is a problem [32,33]. Concerns regarding the incidence of hypospadias following exposure to loratadine led to an investigation by the European Medicines Agency [34]. A causal relationship could neither be confirmed nor excluded with the evidence available and until further investigation has taken place, loratadine should be used with caution in pregnancy. Insufficient data are currently available to assess the safety of fexofenadine, levocetirizine or desloratadine in pregnancy.

Pain and the use of analgesics in pregnancy

Used with caution, the WHO analgesic ladder is applicable for use for treating pain during the first two trimesters of pregnancy. We have commented below on commonly used analgesics.

Paracetamol

Paracetamol is used widely at all stages in pregnancy for relief of pain and as an antipyretic. Its short-term use during pregnancy has not been associated with congenital defects when taken in normal therapeutic doses. A recent study suggested that frequent use of paracetamol between 20 and 32 weeks of pregnancy was associated with an increased risk of asthma in a sub-group of children aged 6–7 years [35,36]. Methodological limitations mean that the findings should be interpreted with caution, and at present paracetamol remains the first-line drug of choice for mild to moderate pain at all stages in pregnancy.

Aspirin

Aspirin is also taken widely in pregnancy. In high doses, it has been shown to be teratogenic in animal studies, while there is controversy about the risk in human pregnancy [37]. Aspirin has a number of undesirable actions in the pregnant woman, principally in late pregnancy. In analgesic doses, it increases the risk of maternal or neonatal bleeding by virtue of its anti-platelet effect [38]. Prolonged use may lead to closure of the ductus arteriosus in utero by inhibiting prostaglandin synthetase. Also, it may delay the onset of labour and increase its duration [39]. For these reasons, analgesic doses of aspirin are best avoided in the third trimester of pregnancy. In contrast, low-dose aspirin (which has been used in the prevention of pregnancy-induced hypertension and pre-eclampsia) appears not to cause adverse effects [40].

Non-steroidal anti-inflammatory drugs

Non-steroidal anti-inflammatory drugs (NSAIDs) have not been linked with congenital defects, but they are best avoided in the periconceptional period as implantation of the blastocyst may be inhibited [41]. These drugs have a similar, although not identical, mode of action to aspirin, and inhibition of prostaglandin synthetase in the fetus may lead to closure of the ductus arteriosus in utero, leading to pulmonary hypertension. Therefore, use of NSAIDs should be avoided in the third trimester if possible, although the effect on the ductus is probably more likely after 34 weeks of gestation. Also, at term, NSAIDs may increase the risk of bleeding because of their effects on platelets. In addition, use of NSAIDs during pregnancy has been reported to cause reversible oligohydramnios as a consequence of reducing fetal urine output [42]. If NSAIDs are considered essential during pregnancy, it is logical to use well-established drugs, such as ibuprofen, diclofenac or indometacin, for which there are most data. Consideration may be given to the use of topical agents such as rubefacients or NSAIDs if appropriate.

Experience is lacking in the use of COX-2 inhibitors in pregnancy, although animal studies have not shown an embryonic risk. In common with non-selective NSAIDs, these agents can cause premature closure of the ductus arteriosus. Currently they are not recommended at any stage in pregnancy.

Opioid analgesics

Much of the data relating to the safety of opioid analgesics in pregnancy have been gathered from studies of women misusing opioids. Such substances are often adulterated, and opiate misusers may inadvertently use mixtures with other drugs. Two American surveillance projects (Michigan Medicaid and Collaborative Perinatal Project) have not recorded an excess rate of congenital defects associated with the use of morphine, pethidine, fentanyl, hydromorphone, oxycodone or methadone [12]. Several published studies have identified a possible increase in malformations associated with the use of codeine [18,43,44]. Nevertheless, extensive experience suggests that the drug is reasonably safe in pregnancy [29].

The principal concern in regular opioid users during pregnancy is that the newborn infant is often opioid dependent. To prevent withdrawal reactions, these babies require slow weaning from opioids and 'quiet' nursing during the postpartum period.

We are not aware of published evidence of the safety of tramadol in early pregnancy, although the British National Formulary (BNF) notes that it has been found to be embryotoxic in animal studies [45]. The drug has been used during labour, with no reports of adverse effect on the neonate [46].

Migraine

Migraine is one disorder that often improves during pregnancy, especially during the second and third trimesters [47]. On the grounds of safety, the drug of first choice is paracetamol. NSAIDs, such as ibuprofen, are possible alternatives but are less desirable for the reasons given above. Ergot alkaloids, such as ergotamine, are uterotonic and are best avoided during pregnancy [48]. Of the serotonin agonists, most experience exists for sumatriptan, and the data suggest it can be used where there is a compelling need [49]. The newer drugs in this class should be used with caution, although no data exist to suggest an increased risk. If drug control of nausea is considered essential, antihistamine antiemetics such as cyclizine or promethazine should be considered; if necessary, occasional doses of prochlorperazine or metoclopramide are probably of low risk, particularly during the second and third trimesters.

Some women will be taking prophylactic treatments for migraine when they become pregnant and may wish to continue treatment during pregnancy. There are data to support the use of β-blockers, particularly propranolol and metoprolol during pregnancy [49]. Nevertheless, a review of continued need should be undertaken in second and third trimesters and should be ideally stopped before delivery because of the potential for adverse effects on fetal heart rate and hypoglycaemia in the newborn infant. There is also much experience of the use of tricyclic antidepressants, such as amitryptyline, in pregnancy and these may be continued until the third trimester when the risk of withdrawal symptoms in the newborn infant must be considered against continued benefit to the mother. There is little data to support the use of pizotifen in pregnancy, although the manufacturer suggests it may be used in compelling circumstances where control has not been achieved with other regimens [50].

Common fungal infections

Candida

Vaginal infections with candida are a common cause of discomfort during pregnancy. Topical agents such as clotrimazole, which have low systemic absorption, are considered to be without significant risk. A recent systematic review of treatment of vaginal candidiasis in pregnancy concluded that imidazoles such as clotrimazole and econazole were more effective than nystatin and that treatment for 7 days may be necessary [51]. Systemic treatment is probably less desirable. There have been reports of congenital malformations in women who took regular, high doses of oral fluconazole in the first trimester of pregnancy for ongoing fungal infections such as coccoidiomycosis [52]. There are less data available on exposure to intermittent or single dose use of the drug, as is likely for vaginal candidiasis. One prescription event monitoring study recorded the outcome of pregnancy in women who had taken either a single 150-mg dose of fluconazole (275 women), several 50-mg doses (3 women) or multiple 150-mg doses (11 women) either during or shortly before becoming pregnant [53]. No abnormalities were identified in those who had taken fluconazole in early pregnancy. Another prospective study concluded that exposure to single doses or short courses of fluconazole during the first trimester did not appear to increase the incidence of congenital defect [54]. A further study has confirmed these findings, in addition reporting no evidence of increased risk of preterm delivery or low birth weight in the pregnancies studied [55]. Although these data are reassuring, fluconazole is clearly best avoided during pregnancy and inadvertent exposure to intermittent or low doses should not be a cause for concern. Itraconazole and ketoconazole are chemically related to fluconazole and are also taken by mouth. Several reports have linked these drugs to congenital malformations [12], and they should be avoided.

Fungal skin infections

Topical imidazoles, such as clotrimazole, can be used to treat most fungal skin infections in pregnancy. Topical treatments are not usually effective for fungal nail infections, but on current evidence, systemic treatments should be avoided in pregnancy. In particular, griseofulvin has been found to be both embryotoxic and teratogenic in some animal species [12]. Less data are available for terbinafine; although animal studies have not found adverse effects on the fetus [56]. Nevertheless, we would suggest avoiding the drug in pregnancy unless absolutely necessary.

Common infestations

Head lice and threadworms are two infestations that women with school-age children may find difficult to control. Also, scabies is not uncommon in young adults. These conditions are discussed below.

Head lice

Head lice (*Pediculus capitis*) have a life cycle of some 40 days, although the infestation has often been established for several months before being detected. The usual treatment involves topical application of one of four insecticides: phenothrin, permethrin, malathion or carbaryl. However, combing with a fine-toothed comb has also been found to be effective (for details see Livingstone

[57]) and 'Bug Buster®' kits can be provided using FP10 prescriptions in the UK.

Many primary care organisations in the UK have a mosaic policy for head lice treatments in order to try to minimise the development of resistance, but it is important to consider the most appropriate choices in pregnancy. One of the first-line drugs in treating head lice is malathion, because there has been more experience with this drug than with newer preparations. Although it is an anticholinesterase, it can be metabolised by the pregnant woman if absorbed systemically, thus limiting exposure of the fetus to the drug. Alternatively, a dimeticone-containing preparation (Hedrin®) is now available which acts as a physical inhibitor fully encapsulating the lice. As it is not absorbed and does not contain a traditional insecticide it can be considered suitable for use by pregnant women [58]. There is now enough experience with pyrethroids, such as permethrin and phenothrin, for these to be used as second-line agents. Aqueous topical preparations are preferable to alcoholic formulations because systemic absorption may be lower. If an insecticide is used in a pregnant woman, intensive combing with a detection comb for 1–2 weeks after treatment may help avoid reinfestation from lice, which hatch from eggs unaffected by treatment. This may help avoid a subsequent course of treatment. Contacts should be treated for head lice only if they have evidence of infestation.

Scabies

Scabies (*Sarcoptes scabiei*) are parasites that burrow under the skin and cause intense pruritis, which is often worse at night. They are spread by close personal contact. Many of the drugs used for head lice are effective against scabies. However, given the considerations outlined above, the treatment of choice in pregnancy is an aqueous preparation of malathion, with pyrethroids being second-line treatments. This should be applied topically to the whole body, excluding the head and neck. Pruritis takes some time to resolve after treatment, and therefore a sedative antihistamine, such as chlorphenamine, may be helpful at night.

Threadworms

Threadworms (*Enterobius vermicularis*) develop in the gastrointestinal tract from ingested eggs. Female worms may then emerge onto the perianal skin to lay eggs, often at night. Pruritis occurs and scratching of the area allows eggs to be transferred to the fingernails. Reinfestation, or spread to other people, may then occur. Non-pharmacological treatment involves hygiene measures aimed to break the cycle of reinfestation. These include a bath or shower in the morning to remove eggs, scrubbing nails, strict hand-washing before handling food, frequent changing of bed linen and wearing of close-fitting pants at night. This is the most desirable method of controlling the problem in pregnant women, particularly in the first trimester of pregnancy. Other members of the household can be treated at the same time with antihelminthics.

Simple hygiene measures sometimes prove ineffective, and medication may be necessary if the worms are causing significant problems with pruritis. Unfortunately, data relating to safety of the two commonly used agents, mebendazole and piperazine, are relatively sparse. Mebendazole is known to be teratogenic in rats, and although it is only poorly absorbed from the gastrointestinal tract in humans, manufacturers state that its use is contraindicated in pregnancy [59]. Piperazine has not been reported to be teratogenic in animals, but it is systemically absorbed to a greater extent than mebendazole. The use of either mebendazole or piperazine is best avoided, particularly in the first trimester. Nevertheless, women who have taken these drugs inadvertently may be reassured that the risks to the fetus are low [60].

Inadvertent drug use in pregnancy

It is not uncommon for a woman to have taken a drug for a minor illness and then to discover that she is pregnant. This shows the importance of judicious prescribing (and medicine taking) for all women with childbearing potential. In many cases it is possible to base advice on information from data sheets and publications such as the BNF [45]. However, it is worth noting that the National Teratology Information Service at Newcastle-upon-Tyne, UK, can often advise in cases of uncertainty (see Appendix 4 of current BNF for phone number). They have access to a considerable body of knowledge relating to outcome of pregnancy for a relatively large number of drugs and follow-up exposure to drugs where current data are limited, in order to provide a more informed response to future enquirers. Thus, in cases of inadvertent drug taking, it is usually possible for health care workers to obtain reasonably sound information on risks to the fetus and the pregnant woman.

References

1 Seto A, Einarson T, Koren G. Pregnancy outcome following first trimester exposure to antihistamines – metaanalysis. *Am J Perinatol* 1997;**14**:119–24.

2 Nelson-Piercy C. Treatment of nausea and vomiting. *Drug Saf* 1998;**19**:155–64.

3 Jewell D, Young G. Interventions for nausea and vomiting in early pregnancy. The Cochrane Database of Systematic Reviews 2003;Issue 4:Art No CD000145.

4 Scialli A, van Tonningen RM. Antiemetics and hyperemesis gravidarum. In: Schaefer C (ed.), *Drugs During Pregnancy and Lactation*. Amsterdam: Elsevier Science; 2001.

5 Baron TH, Ramirez B, Richter JE. Gastrointestinal motility disorders during pregnancy. *Ann Intern Med* 1993;**118**:366–75.

6 Van Thiel DH, Gavaler JS, Stremple J. Heartburn of pregnancy. *Gastroenterology* 1977;**72**:666–8.

7 Ranchet G, Gangemi O, Petrone M. Sucralfate in the treatment of gravidic pyrosis. *G Ital Ostericia Ginecol* 1990;**12**:1–16.

8 Parker S, Schade RR, Pohl CR, et al. Prenatal and neonatal exposure of male rat pups to cimetidine but not ranitidine adversely affects subsequent adult sexual functioning. *Gastroenterology* 1984;**86**:675–80.

9 Garbis H, Elefant E, Diav-Citrin O, et al. Pregnancy outcome after exposure to ranitidine and other H_2-blockers. A collaborative study of the European Network of Teratology Information Services. *Reprod Toxicol* 2005;**19**:453–8.

10 Broussard CN, Richter JE. Treating gastro-oesophageal reflux disease during pregnancy and lactation: what are the safest therapy options? *Drug Saf* 1998;**19**:325–37.

11 Lalkin A, Loebstein R, Addis R, et al. The safety of omeprazole during pregnancy: a multicenter prospective controlled study. *Am J Obstet Gynecol* 1998;**179**:727–30.

12 Briggs GG, Freeman RK, Yaffe SJ. *Drugs in Pregnancy and Lactation, 7th edition*. Baltimore: Lippinott, Williams & Wilkins; 2005.

13 Wyeth Pharmaceuticals. Summary of product characteristics for Zoton® (lansoprazole). Available at: http://www.emc.medicines.org. uk/. Accessed 22 January 2006.

14 Hedgley CA, McElhatton PR, Thomas SHL. Outcome of pregnancy following maternal treatment with proton pump inhibitors (PPIs). *Clin Toxicol* 2005;**43**:431.

15 Rost van Tonningen M. Gastrointestinal and antilipidemic agents and spasmolytics. In: Schaefer C (ed.), *Drugs During Pregnancy and Lactation*. Amsterdam: Elsevier Science; 2001.

16 Lee A, Schofield S. Drug use in pregnancy: 2. Common medical problems. *Pharm J* 1994;**252**:57–60.
17 Siebert JR, Barr M, Jr, Jackson JC, Benjamin DR. Ebsteins anomaly and extracardiac effects. *Am J Dis Child* 1989;**143**:570–2.
18 Heinonen OP, Slone D, Shapiro S. *Birth Defects and Drugs in Pregnancy*. Littleton, MA: Publishing Sciences Group; 1977.
19 Einarson A, Mastroiacovo P, Arnon J, et al. Prospective, controlled, multicentre study of loperamide in pregnancy. *Can J Gastroenterol* 2000;**14**: 185–7.
20 Alonso-Coello P, Guyatt G, Heels-Ansdell D, et al. Laxatives for the treatment of hemorrhoids. The Cochrane Database of Systematic Reviews 2005;Issue 4:Art No CD004649.
21 Arroll B, Kenealy T. Antibiotics for the common cold and acute purulent rhinitis. The Cochrane Database of Systematic Reviews 2005;Issue 3:Art No CD000247.
22 Williams JW, Aguilar C, Cornell J, et al. Antibiotics for acute maxillary sinusitis. The Cochrane Database of Systematic Reviews 2003;Issue 2:Art No CD000243.
23 Del Mar CB, Glasziou PP, Spinks AB. Antibiotics for sore throat. The Cochrane Database of Systematic Reviews 2004;Issue 2:Art No CD000023.
24 Singh M. Heated, humidified air for the common cold. The Cochrane Database of Systematic Reviews 2004; Issue 2:Art No CD001728.
25 Taverner D, Latte J, Draper M. Nasal decongestants for the common cold. The Cochrane Database of Systematic Reviews 2004; Issue 3:Art No CD001953.
26 Schroeder K, Fahey T. Over-the-counter medications for acute cough in children and adults in ambulatory settings. The Cochrane Database of Systematic Reviews 2004;Issue 4:Art No CD001831.
27 Werler MM, Mitchell AA, Hernandez-Diaz S, Honein MA. Use of over-the-counter medications during pregnancy. *Am J Obstet Gynecol* 2005;**193**:771–7.
28 Dykes MHM. Evaluation of an antiasthmatic agent cromolyn sodium (Aarane, Intal). *JAMA* 1974;**227**:1061–2.
29 Lee A. Common problems in pregnancy. In: Lee A, Inch S, Finnigan D (eds.), *Therapeutics in Pregnancy and Lactation*. Oxford: Radcliffe; 2000.
30 Anonymous. Any place for depot triamcinolone in hay fever? *Drug and Ther Bull* 1999;**37**(3):17–18.
31 Schatz M, Pettiti D. Antihistamines and pregnancy. *Ann Allerg Asthma Immunol* 1997;**78**:157–9.
32 Einarson A, Bailey B, Jung G, et al. Prospective controlled study of hydroxyzine and cetirizine in pregnancy. *Ann Allerg Asthma Immunol* 1997;**78**:183–6.

33 Rost van Tonningen M. Antiallergy drugs and desensitisation. In: Schaefer C (ed.), *Drugs During Pregnancy and Lactation*. Amsterdam: Elsevier Science; 2001.
34 European Medicines Agency (EMEA). Report on Loratadine 28th April 2004: CPMP/1333/03. Available at: http://www.emea.eu.int/pdfs/human/referral/loratadine/133303en.pdf/. Accessed 22 January 2006.
35 Shaheen SO, Newson RB, Sherriff A, et al. Paracetamol use pregnancy and wheezing in early childhood. *Thorax* 2002;**57**:958–63.
36 Shaheen SO, Newson RB, Henderson AJ, et al. Prenatal paracetamol exposure and risk of asthma and elevated IgE in childhood. *Clin Exp Allergy Rev* 2005;**35**:18–25.
37 Reprorisk database. In: *Drugdex information system (exp. 03/99)*. Denver, CO: Micromedex Inc.; 1999.
38 Stuart MJ, Gross SJ, Elrad H, Graeber JE. Effects of acetylsalicylic acid ingestion on maternal and neonatal haemostasis. *N Engl J Med* 1982;**307**:902–12.
39 Lewis RN, Schulman D. Influence of acetylsalicylic acid, an inhibitor of prostaglandin synthesis on the duration of human gestation and labour. *Lancet* 1973;**2**:1159–61.
40 CLASP Collaborative Group. Low dose aspirin in pregnancy and early childhood development: follow-up of the collaborative aspirin study in pregnancy. *Br J Obstet Gynaecol* 1995;**102**:861–8.
41 Dawood MY. Nonsteroidal antiinflammatory drugs and reproduction. *Am J Obstet Gynecol* 1993;**169**:1255–65.
42 Hickok DE, Hollenbach KA, Reilley SF, Nyberg DA. The association between decreased amniotic fluid volume and treatment with nonsteroidal anti-inflammatory agents for preterm labour. *Am J Obstet Gynecol* 1989;**160**:1525–31.
43 Bracken M, Holford TR. Exposure to prescribed drugs in pregnancy and association with congenital malformations. *Obstet Gynecol* 1981;**58**:336–44.
44 Saxen I. Epidemiology of cleft lip and palate: an attempt to rule out chance correlations. *Br J Prev Soc Med* 1975;**29**:103–10.
45 Joint Formulary Committee. *British National Formulary, 50th edition*. London: British Medical Association and Royal Pharmaceutical Society of Great Britain; 2005.
46 Viegas OA, Khaw B, Ratnam SS. Tramadol in labour pain in primiparous patients. A prospective comparative clinical trial. *Eur J Obstet Gynecol Reprod Biol* 1993;**49**:131–5.
47 Uknis A, Silberstein SD. Review article: migraine and pregnancy. *Headache* 1991;**31**:372–4.
48 Pfaffenrath V, Rehm M. Migraine in pregnancy. What are the safest treatment options? *Drug Saf* 1998;**19**:383–8.

49 Reuvers M. Analgesics and antiphlogistics. In: Schaefer C (ed.), *Drugs During Pregnancy and Lactation*. Amsterdam: Elsevier Science; 2001.

50 Novartis. Datasheet for Sanomigran® (pizotifen). Available at: http://www.emc.medicines.org.uk/. Accessed 31 July 2006.

51 Young GL, Jewell D. Topical treatment for vaginal candidiasis (thrush) in pregnancy. The Cochrane Database of Systematic Reviews 2001; Issue 4: Art No CD000225.

52 Pursley TJ, Blomquist IK, Abraham J, Andersen HF, Bartley JA. Fluconazole-induced congenital anomalies in three infants. *Clin Infect Dis* 1996;**22**:336–40.

53 Inman WH, Pearce G, Wilton L. Safety of fluconazole in the treatment of vaginal candidiasis. A prescription-event monitoring study, with special reference to the outcome of pregnancy. *Eur J Clin Pharmacol* 1994;**46**: 115–8.

54 Mastriacovo P, Mazzone T, Botto LD, et al. Prospective assessment of pregnancy outcomes after first trimester exposure to fluconazole. *Am J Obstet Gynecol* 1996;**9**:1645–50.

55 Sorensen HT, Nielsen GL, Olesen C, et al. Risk of malformations and other outcomes in children exposed to fluconazole in utero. *Br J Clin Pharmacol* 1999;**48**:234–8.

56 Novartis. Datasheet for Lamasil® (terbinafine). Available at: http:// www.emc.medicines.org.uk/. Accessed 22 January 2006.

57 Livingstone C. Lice and scabies. *Pharm J* 1998;**260**:204–6.

58 Burgess IF, Brown CM, Lee PN. Treatment of head louse infestation with dimeticone lotion: randomised controlled equivalence trial. *BMJ* 2005;**330**:1423–5.

59 Janssen-Cilag Ltd. Datasheet for mebendazole (Vermox) tablets. Available at: http://www.emc.medicines.org.uk/. Accessed 22 January 2006.

60 Leach F. Management of threadworm infestation during pregnancy. *Arch Dis Child* 1990;**65**:399–40.

CHAPTER 3
Antibiotics in pregnancy

Tim Weller, Conor Jamieson

Key points

- There is little evidence regarding the safety of most antimicrobial therapy in pregnancy
- Clinical experience indicates the safety of penicillins and cephalosporins
- Serious infections in pregnancy should be treated aggressively

Introduction

The use of antimicrobial agents during pregnancy often needs to be considered as pregnant women are at the same risk of acquiring infectious diseases as anyone else. Indeed, they may be more prone to certain infections, such as those of the urinary tract. In some cases, such as asymptomatic bacteriuria, therapy is primarily required to prevent fetal loss [1] rather than for the treatment of the mother. Regardless of who is the main beneficiary, it is important to know which compounds can be used with minimal risk in minor infections and to have some appreciation of the balance of risks for more serious cases.

When the risk to the fetus is being assessed, several points should be considered. With many antimicrobial agents, we now have more than 40 years of experience of freedom from congenital abnormality. The results of studies performed in animals should be viewed with caution. Sulphonamides, for example, can cause gross fetal malformations when given in high doses to rats and mice [2], but teratogenicity has not been recorded in humans despite use

Prescribing in Pregnancy, 4th edition. Edited by Peter Rubin and Margaret Ramsay,
 ISBN: 978-1-4051-4712-5.

for more than 50 years. One of the reasons why laboratory animals make poor models for studying fetal damage is the profound effect antibiotics have on their normal gastrointestinal flora and consequently on the animal's metabolism.

There are some drugs, however, with proven toxicity in humans, which should definitely be avoided. Streptomycin, for example, has caused neonatal ototoxicity after long-term treatment of tuberculosis [3,4]. By implication, the other aminoglycosides such as gentamicin, tobramycin, netilmicin and amikacin should be avoided for minor infections, although there is no hard evidence that they cause the same problem.

Changes in the dynamics of blood flow and other physiological effects of pregnancy can influence the pharmacokinetics of many drugs. Philipson showed that serum concentrations of ampicillin in women who were 9–36 weeks pregnant were half the values found in the same women when they were not pregnant [5]. Low maternal concentrations have been described after the ingestion of many antimicrobial agents, although the therapeutic implications of this are difficult to assess.

Failure of antibiotic treatment may be blamed incorrectly on the wrong choice of antibiotic, and the drug might be replaced with a potentially more toxic agent. This could be particularly dangerous when concern for the fetus prevents the doctor from giving high doses whilst treating a serious infection in the mother. In general, full adult doses should be used when treating infection in a pregnant woman. Similarly, the length of therapy should be dictated by the disease and not unduly influenced by the fact that the patient is pregnant. Inadequate treatment, which may be followed by further courses of antibiotics, is likely to put the mother and fetus at greater risk than a full course of the appropriate drug.

Antimicrobial agents

Table 3.1 lists most antimicrobial agents available in the UK together with their possible toxic effects on the fetus during pregnancy. Each is given a safety rating:

'Probably safe' – controlled studies in women fail to demonstrate a risk to the fetus in the first trimester or later trimesters. A first-choice drug if an antimicrobial agent has to be used.

'Caution' – there are no controlled studies in pregnant women and studies in animals have not demonstrated a risk to the

Table 3.1 Antimicrobial agents and their possible adverse effects

		Adverse effects on fetus		
Agent	**Use**	**First trimester**	**Second and third trimester**	**Comments**
Penicillins				
Phenoxymethylpenicillin, penicillin G and long-acting penicillins	Probably safe		Allergy; possibility of sensitising the fetus	No adverse effects recorded during decades of use
Ampicillin and amoxicillin	Probably safe		Allergy; possibility of sensitising the fetus	No adverse effects recorded during decades of use
Ampicillin pro-drugs (talampicillin, pivampicillin, bacampicillin)	Probably safe		Allergy; possibility of sensitising the fetus	Limited data; no adverse effects recorded
Co-amoxiclav	Probably safe		Allergy; possibility of sensitising the fetus	Limited data; no adverse effects recorded
Ticarcillin, piperacillin/tazobactam and other antipseudomonal penicillins	Probably safe		Allergy; possibility of sensitising the fetus	No adverse effects recorded during decades of use
Flucloxacillin and other antistaphylococcal penicillins	Probably safe		Allergy; possibility of sensitising the fetus	No adverse effects recorded during decades of use

Cephalosporins			
Oral (cefalexin, cefadroxil, cefradine, cefaclor, cefixime, cefpodoxime, cefprozil, cefuroxime)	Probably safe	Allergy; possibility of sensitising the fetus	Limited data; no adverse effects recorded
Intravenous (cefuroxime, ceftazidime, cefotaxime, ceftriaxone, cefpirome, cefoxitin)	Probably safe	Allergy; possibility of sensitising the fetus	Limited data; no adverse effects recorded
Carbapenems			
Imipenem	Avoid		Toxicity in animals
Meropenem, ertapenem	Caution		Limited data; use only if benefit outweighs risk
Other β-lactams			
Aztreonam	Caution		Limited data; use only if benefit outweighs risk
Mecillinam	Probably safe		
Macrolides/lincosamides			
Erythromycin	Probably safe		No adverse effects recorded during decades of use
Azithromycin, clarithromycin	Caution		Limited data; alternatives are usually available
Clindamycin	Probably safe		Beware of maternal pseudomembranous colitis

(*Continued*)

Table 3.1 (*Continued*)

Agent	Use	Adverse effects on fetus		Comments
		First trimester	Second and third trimester	
Tetracyclines				
Tetracycline, demeclocycline, doxycycline, lymecycline, minocycline, oxytetracycline	Avoid	Effect on development in animals	Discolouration and dysplasia of bones and teeth, cataracts	Possible maternal hepatotoxicity
Aminoglycosides				
Amikacin, gentamicin, neomycin, netilmicin, tobramycin	Caution		Theoretical risk of ototoxicity	Use in serious sepsis if benefit outweighs risk
Quinolones				
Ciprofloxacin, levofloxacin, moxifloxacin, nalidixic acid, norfloxacin, ofloxacin	Avoid	Arthropathy in animal studies	Arthropathy in animal studies	May be used if no alternative available
Other antibacterial agents				
Chloramphenicol	Avoid	No evidence of adverse effects to the fetus in early pregnancy, but a safer alternative is usually available	Grey baby syndrome	Safe if given topically as absorption is minimal

Colistin	Avoid		Possible fetal toxicity	
Fusidic acid	Probably safe			Limited data; no adverse effects recorded
Metronidazole, tinidazole	Probably safe	Theoretical teratogenic risk		No adverse effects recorded, confirmed by meta-analysis
Nitrofurantion	Caution		Risk of haemolysis at term	Safe, except during labour and delivery
Vancomycin, teicoplanin	Caution			Limited data; use only if benefits outweigh risk
Trimethoprim	Caution	Theoretical teratogenic risk		No adverse events recorded; use if benefits outweigh risk
Co-trimoxazole	Avoid	Theoretical teratogenic risk	Neonatal haemolysis and methaemoglobinaemia	
Antituberculous agents				
Capreomycin	Caution			Use only if benefits outweigh risk; teratogenic in animal studies
Cycloserine	Caution			Use only if benefit outweighs risk
Rifampicin	Caution	Teratogenic at high doses in animals	Possible increased risk of neonatal bleeding	Use only if benefit outweighs risk; vitamin K should be given to mother and neonate; avoid in mothers with liver disease

(Continued)

Table 3.1 *(Continued)*

Agent	Use	Adverse effects on fetus		
		First trimester	Second and third trimester	Comments
Isoniazid	Probably safe			
Ethambutol	Caution	Teratogenic in animals		No adverse effects reported but teratogenic in animals
Pyrazinamide	Caution			Limited data; use only when benefit outweighs risk
Streptomycin	Avoid		Ototoxicity	Safer agents always available
Antifungal agents				
Amphotericin	Caution			Limited data; use only if benefit outweighs risk
Caspofungin	Caution	Toxicity in animal studies		Use only if benefit outweighs risk
Fluconazole	Caution			Limited data; toxicity at high doses in animals; use only if benefit outweighs risk
Itraconazole, ketoconazole	Avoid	Teratogenic in animals		
Miconazole, clotrimazole	Caution			Absorbed from vaginal topical use, but no adverse effects recorded

Flucytosine	Avoid	Teratogenic in animals	
Terbinafine	Caution		Limited data; treatment may be postponed until after pregnancy
Griesofulvin	Avoid	Fetotoxic and teratogenic	Women should avoid pregnancy for 1 mo following treatment
Nystatin	Probably safe		Minimal absorption
Voriconazole	Caution		Use only if benefit outweighs risk; toxicity in animal studies
Antiparasitic agents			
Albendazole, mebendazole, thiabendazole	Avoid	Teratogenic in animals	
Atovaquone	Caution		Limited data; use if benefit outweighs risk
Piperazine	Probably safe		Limited data; treatment may be postponed until after pregnancy
Pentamidine	Caution		Limited experience; use if benefit outweighs risk
Antiviral agents			
Aciclovir, famciclovir, valaciclovir	Caution		Limited data; use if benefit outweighs risk

(Continued)

Table 3.1 (*Continued*)

Agent	Use	Adverse effects on fetus		Comments
		First trimester	**Second and third trimester**	
Cidofovir	Avoid	Teratogenic in animals		
Ganciclovir, valganciclovir	Avoid	Teratogenic in animals		
Foscarnet	Avoid			Manufacturer advises avoidance in pregnancy
Adefovir	Caution			Toxicity in animal studies; use only if benefit outweighs risk
Amantadine	Avoid	Embryotoxic in animals		
Oseltamavir, zanamavir	Caution			Limited data available; use only if benefit outweighs risk
Anti-HIV agents				
Nucleoside reverse transcriptase inhibitors				
Abacavir	Avoid			Toxicity in animal studies; manufacturer recommends avoidance in pregnancy
Lamivudine	Caution			Manufacturer recommends avoidance during first trimester

Didanosine, emtricitabine, stavudine, tenofovir, zalcitabine	Caution	Zalcitabine is teratogenic in animals		Limited data; use if benefit outweighs risk
Zidovudine	Probably safe			Treatment during pregnancy reduces risk of congenital infection
Protease inhibitors				
Amprenavir, atazanavir, lopinavir, nelfinavir, ritonavir, saquinavir	Caution		Atazanavir may cause neonatal hyperbilirubinaemia at term	Limited data; use if benefit outweighs risk; high propylene glycol content in some oral solutions
Indinavir	Caution		Theoretical risk of neonatal hyperbilirubinaemia and renal stones if used at term	Toxicity in animal studies; use only if benefit outweighs risk
Non-nucleoside reverse transcriptase inhibitors				
Efavirenz	Caution			Toxicity in animal studies; use only if benefit outweighs risk
Nevirapine	Caution			Use if benefit outweighs risk
Other antiretrovirals				
Enfuvirtide	Caution			Use if benefit outweighs risk

Table 3.2 Infections in pregnancy with recommended treatment

Condition	First-choice treatment	Second-choice treatment	Comments
Asymptomatic bacteriuria or simple cystitis	Nitrofurantion (except at term), co-amoxiclav or cefalexin by mouth	Ampicillin or amoxicillin, pivmecillinam	Seven days for asymptomatic bacteriuria, 3 days for cystitis
Acute pyelonephritis	Cefuroxime or co-amoxiclav intravenously		Treat for 7–10 days but may switch to oral when apyrexial for 24 h
Pharyngitis	Phenoxymethylpenicillin by mouth or benzylpenicillin intravenously	Erythromycin	Antibiotics usually unnecessary as 70–80% caused by viruses
Sinusitis	Amoxicillin or co-amoxiclav		Antibiotics often unnecessary
Chest infection (mild)	Amoxicillin (+ erythromycin if atypicals suspected) by mouth	Erythromycin	As per British Thoracic Society recommendations [6]
Chest infection (severe)	Cefuroxime (+ erythromycin if atypicals suspected) intravenously		As per British Thoracic Society recommendations [6]
Tuberculosis	Rifampicin, isoniazid, pyrazinamide and ethambutol	Seek expert advice as many agents may be teratogenic	As per British Thoracic Society recommendations [7]
Skin/soft tissue/wound infection	Flucloxacillin	Clindamycin	

Bacterial vaginosis	Metronidazole by mouth	Metronidazole or clindamycin intravaginal gel/cream or clindamycin by mouth	
Gonorrhoea	Ceftriaxone intramuscularly or cefixime by mouth	Intramuscular spectinomycin	
Syphilis	Intramuscular procaine penicillin G	Seek expert advice	
Chlamydia trachomatis	Erythromycin	Amoxicillin	
Pelvic inflammatory disease	Intramuscular ceftriaxone + intravenous/oral erythromycin ± oral metronidazole if severe disease		
Listeriosis	Amoxicillin or ampicillin	Add intravenous gentamicin if severe disease	
Endocarditis Streptococcal	Benzylpenicillin + gentamicin		For full details see British Society for Antimicrobial Chemotherapy guidelines [8]
Staphylococcal	Flucloxacillin + gentamicin		
Meningitis	Benzylpenicillin	Cefotaxime or ceftriaxone	
Serious undiagnosed sepsis	Cefuroxime/cefotaxime ± gentamicin ± metronidazole		

fetus, or else animal studies have shown an adverse effect that has not been confirmed in controlled studies in women in the first or later trimesters. These agents should only be given if the potential benefit outweighs the risk.

'Avoid' – indicates that the agent carries evidence of fetal risk in humans. It should only be used in life-threatening infections where no other drug is suitable.

Treatment and prevention of specific infections

Table 3.2 lists some of the common infections encountered in pregnancy. The agents recommended are for empirical therapy and are based on the pathogens most likely to cause each infection. It is particularly important to take cultures from pregnant patients *before* treatment so that a safe and efficacious change can be made if the patient does not respond or if the causative organism proves resistant to initial therapy.

The first choice of treatment is usually an agent listed as 'probably safe' in Table 3.1, although not necessarily so. A second choice may be used if the patient is allergic to the first compound or the bacteria responsible for the infection are resistant to it. Where one antibiotic is significantly better than all other therapies, it may be recommended despite the need for caution when prescribing in pregnancy. Some of the conditions are not seen frequently enough in pregnancy for any suitable agent to be regarded as unequivocally safe. In such cases the problem has been highlighted in the table, but specialist advice should be sought from an expert in the field before embarking on treatment. Finally, if an infection needs treating then it needs treating properly and so the dose chosen should be that which is normally used for the condition.

Prevention of infection in pregnancy protects both the mother and child. *Prophylaxis* should be given whenever the risk of disease outweighs the risk associated with the agent used to prevent it. Prophylactic regimes recommended in pregnancy are detailed in Table 3.3. In most cases they do not differ from those used for non-pregnant patients.

Urinary tract infection

The most common reason for a pregnant woman to take antibiotics is to treat acute cystitis or asymptomatic bacteriuria. The latter condition is associated with a significant incidence of pyelonephritis

Table 3.3 Antimicrobial prophylaxis in pregnancy

Condition	First-choice prophylaxis	Second-choice prophylaxis	Comments
Endocarditis	Amoxicillin	Clindamycin	As per British Society of Antimicrobial Chemotherapy guidelines [8]
Meningococcal meningitis	Rifampicin	Ceftriaxone intramuscularly	
Surgical prophylaxis			
Clean surgery	No prophylaxis		As per Scottish
Clean-contaminated surgery	Cefuroxime – single dose		Intercollegiate Guidelines Network recommendations [9]
Contaminated surgery	Cefuroxime and metronidazole – one to three doses		
Tuberculosis	Isoniazid		Give pyridoxine supplements with isoniazid

and possibly preterm delivery and low birth weight, making treatment essential [1]. It is recommended that antibiotics are administered for 7 days if bacteriuria is covert, but symptomatic infection usually responds to a shorter, 3 day, course [10]. The first-choice antibiotics would be nitrofurantoin (except during labour and delivery) or a first-generation cephalosporin, such as cefalexin. Amoxicillin is an alternative, if the infecting organism is susceptible, but resistance rates are around 50% in *Escherichia coli* from community-acquired urinary tract infection [11]. Pivmecillinam also has proven efficacy and safety, and very low rates of resistance. The manufacturers of co-amoxiclav still recommend caution, but it does seem to be a safe alternative. Although trimethoprim is theoretically teratogenic during the first trimester, short-term use is unlikely to cause problems.

There are occasions when *Pseudomonas aeruginosa* or other resistant isolates, insensitive to all the oral agents recommended above, are cultured. In these cases, it is important to establish that the organism is truly causing an infection, by repeating urine culture before treatment is undertaken. The patient may then have to receive a potentially harmful antibiotic, such as intramuscular gentamicin, or be admitted to a hospital for administration of a safe intravenous one, such as ceftazidime.

Lower respiratory tract infections

The most common bacterial pathogen of the lower respiratory tract, *Streptococcus pneumoniae,* is usually sensitive to penicillin, amoxicillin and ampicillin. These agents should be the first choice for empirical treatment of a mild community-acquired infection. Another agent, such as co-amoxiclav, may be indicated if culture reveals *Haemophilus influenzae* or if the patient fails to respond. Patients admitted to hospital with severe pulmonary infection can be treated with cefuroxime or cefotaxime according to the British Thoracic Society guidelines [6].

Erythromycin has two indications in community-acquired lower respiratory tract infection:

- To treat 'atypical' pneumonia caused by bacteria such as *Mycoplasma pneumoniae, Chlamydia pneumoniae* and *Legionella pneumophila*
- For oral treatment of penicillin-allergic patients.

In both cases, the newer macrolides azithromycin and clarithromycin are just as effective but they do not have the proven record of safety in pregnancy.

Tuberculosis

Although the possibility of teratogenesis was suspected with both rifampicin and ethambutol, they have been found to be safe in clinical practice. The Joint Tuberculosis Committee of the British Thoracic Society recommends that the treatment of tuberculosis in pregnant women should be no different to that normally given [7]. Of the second-line agents, streptomycin is absolutely contraindicated in pregnancy because of the occurrence of ototoxicity in the fetus [3,4]. Ethionamide and prothionamide should only be used if no other compounds are available as they may be teratogenic.

Infections of the genital tract

The British Association for Sexual Health and HIV produce evidence-based guidelines for the management of sexually transmitted disease (http://www.bashh.org/guidelines/ceguidelines.asp). The following advice is based on these guidelines.

There is conflicting evidence regarding the association of *bacterial vaginosis* with premature delivery. It is recommended that symptomatic pregnant women should be treated in the usual way, with metronidazole. This antibiotic has some theoretical risks but has been found to be safe in clinical practice. Asymptomatic women should not be screened or treated.

Gonorrhoea in pregnancy can be treated using a single dose of intramuscular ceftriaxone 250 mg or oral cefixime 400 mg. If the organism is resistant or the patient is allergic to cephalosporins, then intramuscular spectinomycin 2 g is recommended.

All pregnant women should be screened for syphilis. Treatment should be instituted if early infection is detected as, without it, fetal infection is almost inevitable. The regime in pregnancy, intramuscular procaine penicillin G 750 mg for 10 days, does not differ from standard regimens. Therapy for the penicillin-allergic patient can be difficult because other agents, such as erythromycin, do not reliably treat the unborn child [12]. In such cases expert advice should be sought, as penicillin-desensitisation of the patient may be the best option.

C. trachomatis infection during pregnancy should be treated with oral erythromycin, as doxycycline and ofloxacin are contraindicated. Patients unable to tolerate 500 mg four times a day for 7 days can be given 500 mg twice daily for 2 weeks. Alternatives are amoxicillin, which induces latency in vitro and may be unreliable, or azithromycin, which has not been fully evaluated in pregnancy. A test of cure should be performed 3 weeks after the end of therapy.

Pelvic inflammatory disease is not uncommon in pregnancy and is associated with an increase in both maternal and fetal morbidity. Treatment is difficult as none of the recommended evidence-based regimens are of proven safety in pregnancy. The chosen combination should be based on local sensitivity patterns and may include intramuscular or intravenous ceftriaxone plus oral or intravenous erythromycin, and possibly oral metronidazole in clinically severe disease.

Listeriosis

Infection with *Listeria monocytogenes* during pregnancy usually occurs in the third trimester. Stillbirth ensues in 22% of untreated cases and spontaneous abortion; premature labour or neonatal infection can also occur [13]. Intravenous ampicillin or amoxicillin has been effective for the mother and can prevent fetal damage. In severe maternal infection, it may also be necessary to give gentamicin.

Group B streptococcal colonisation

Group B streptococci are normal inhabitants of the female genital tract and can cause neonatal meningitis and bacteraemia. Although this organism can often be detected throughout pregnancy, treatment of the mother prior to delivery is both ineffective and unnecessary. However, selective administration of benzylpenicillin to high-risk patients has been shown to reduce the incidence of neonatal infection [14]. Intrapartum prophylaxis should be considered if group B streptococci are detected incidentally in the later weeks of pregnancy or if a previous baby has had neonatal group B streptococcal disease [15]. The advised regime is benzylpenicillin 2.4 g 6-hourly until delivery. Intravenous clindamycin 900 mg 8-hourly can be used for penicillin-allergic women.

Serious sepsis

It is rare to have a pregnant patient with serious undiagnosed sepsis. When such a situation does occur, the risk to the mother outweighs any risk to the fetus. Therefore, the most appropriate antibiotics for the patient's condition should be given in full doses. Once a pathogen and its antimicrobial susceptibilities have been identified, treatment can be directed at that organism. A suitable choice for empirical therapy would be a second- or third-generation cephalosporin (cefuroxime or cefotaxime), with the addition of gentamicin and/or metronidazole if this is warranted by the clinical condition. If an aminoglycoside was required, careful monitoring is required to ensure that the patient is receiving sufficient drug, and neither she nor the fetus is being exposed to unacceptably high levels.

HIV

The aims of treatment of HIV infection in pregnancy are to reduce the risk of toxicity to the fetus, to minimise the viral load and disease progression in the mother and to prevent transmission of infection to the neonate. Prophylaxis is currently recommended for all HIV-infected pregnant women to prevent vertical transmission [16]. It has been shown that the rate of HIV transmission from mother to child is significantly reduced if zidovudine is used during pregnancy [17,18]. However, combination therapy with some of the newer agents maximises the chance of preventing transmission as well as provides optimum treatment for the mother. It is generally recommended that women currently receiving therapy for HIV infection should remain on the same drugs during pregnancy [19]. Specialist advice should be sought for the management of such patients.

Toxoplasmosis

A diagnosis of acute toxoplasmosis can be established in the mother by detection of specific IgM or a rise in maternal IgG. Fetal infection can only be confirmed by isolation of parasites from fetal blood. Transmission to the fetus is relatively uncommon in the first trimester, but when cases occur, the disease is severe. In the third trimester, maternal infection is almost always transmitted to the fetus, but most babies will have no overt disease at birth.

Management of toxoplasmosis in pregnancy requires specialist knowledge, and liaison with an expert is advised. Maternal infection can be treated using oral clindamycin 300 mg 6-hourly for 3–4 weeks. If IgM is positive, protect the fetus using oral spiramycin 1 g 8-hourly for the duration of pregnancy.

Surgical prophylaxis

Although elective operations are avoided in pregnancy, emergency operations may be necessary. As in non-pregnant patients, a short course of an appropriate agent is indicated. If there is evidence of established intra-abdominal sepsis, a parenteral cephalosporin such as cefuroxime plus metronidazole should be given. Alternatives include co-amoxiclav or clindamycin. The number of doses, one to three, depends upon the degree of contamination expected (see Table 3.3). If there is proven infection at operation, 3–5-day treatment is required.

The risk of infection following emergency caesarean section is substantial and the need for prophylactic antibiotics is clear. There is a smaller risk after an elective procedure, but most practitioners still give perioperative antibiotics. One dose of cefuroxime, with or without metronidazole, ought to be sufficient, provided it is given early enough to be present in the tissues when the incision is made. Thus, it should be administered before or during induction of anaesthesia. There is no advantage, in fact there is a significant disadvantage, in delaying prophylaxis until after the cord had been clamped.

Vaccination

As a general rule, immunisation during pregnancy should be avoided if possible, although most vaccines are probably safe to give. Particular caution is advised in relation to the live vaccines [20]. Immunisation against rubella is contraindicated during pregnancy and conception should be avoided in the month following administration of the vaccine. Similarly, polio vaccine should not be given in the first 4 months of pregnancy. In circumstances when there is a significant risk of disease, following exposure to hepatitis B positive blood or travel to an area endemic for yellow fever for instance, then the benefit gained by immunisation of the mother may well outweigh the risk to the fetus.

References

1 Condie AP, Brumfitt W, Reeves DS, Williams JD. The effects of bacteriuria in pregnancy on foetal health. In: Brumfitt W, Asscher AW (eds.), *Urinary Tract Infection*. London: Oxford University Press; 1973.
2 Kato T, Kitagawa S. Production of congenital abnormalities in the fetuses of rats and mice with various sulphonamides. *Congenit Abnormal* 1973;**13**:7–15.
3 Assael BM, Parini R, Rusconi F. Ototoxicity of aminoglycoside antibiotics in infants and children. *Pediatr Infect Dis* 1982;**1**:357–67.
4 Conway N, Birt BD. Streptomycin in pregnancy: effect on the foetal ear. *BMJ* 1966;**ii**:260–3.
5 Philipson A. Pharmacokinetics of antibiotics in pregnancy and labour. *Clin Pharmacokinet* 1979;**4**:297–309.
6 The British Thoracic Society. Guidelines for the management of community acquired pneumonia in adults. *Thorax* 2001;**56**(Suppl IV): iv1–64.
7 The Joint Tuberculosis Committee of the British Thoracic Society. Chemotherapy and management of tuberculosis in the United Kingdom: recommendations 1998. *Thorax* 1998;**53**(7):536–48.
8 Eliott TSJ, Foweraker J, Gould FK, et al. Guidelines for the antibiotic treatment of endocarditis in adults: report of the Working Party of the

British Society for Antimicrobial Chemotherapy. *J Antimicrob Chemother* 2004;**54**:971–81.

9 Scottish Intercollegiate Guidelines Network. Antibiotic prophylaxis in surgery. SIGN Publication No. 45, Edinburgh, July 2000.

10 Bint AJ, Hill D. Bacteriuria in pregnancy – an update on significance, diagnosis and management. *J Antimicrob Chemother* 1994;**33**(Suppl A):93–7.

11 Farrell DJ, Morrissey I, De Reubis D, Robbins M, Felmingham D. A UK multicentre study of the antimicrobial sensitivity of bacterial pathogens causing urinary tract infection. *J Infect* 2003;**46**:96–100.

12 Hashisaki P, Wertzberger GG, Conrand GL, Nichols CR. Erythromycin failure in the treatment of syphilis in pregnant women. *Sex Transm Dis* 1983;**10**:36–8.

13 Kalstone C. Successful antepartum treatment of listeriosis. *Am J Obstet Gynecol* 1991;**164**:57–8.

14 Omenaca Teres F, Mattoras R, Garcia Perea A, Elorza MD. Prevention of neonatal group B streptococcal sepsis. *Pediatr Infect Dis J* 1987;**6**:874.

15 Royal College of Obstetricians and Gynaecologists. *Prevention of Early Onset Neonatal Group B Streptococcal Disease*. Guideline Number 36. Available at: www.rcog.org.uk. Accessed November 2003.

16 Minkoff H, Augenbraun M. Antiretroviral therapy for pregnant women. *Am J Obstet Gynecol* 1997;**176**:478–89.

17 Connor EM, Sperling RS, Gelber R, et al. Reduction of maternal-infant transmission of human immunodeficiency virus type 1 with zidovudine treatment. *NEJM* 1994;**331**:1173–80.

18 Lallemant M, Jourdain G, Le Coeur S, et al. A trial of shortened zidovudine regimens to prevent mother-to-child transmission of human immunodeficiency virus type I. *NEJM* 2000;**343**:982–91.

19 British HIV Association. Guidelines for the management of HIV infection in pregnant women and the prevention of mother-to-child transmission of HIV. Available at: www.bhiva.org. Accessed 31 March 2005.

20 Salisbury DM, Begg NT (eds.). *Immunisation Against Infectious Disease*. London: HMSO; 1996.

CHAPTER 4
Anticoagulants in pregnancy

Bethan Myers

Introduction

Anticoagulants are used for an increasing number of clinical situations in pregnancy. These include prophylaxis and treatment of venous thromboembolic disease, prophylaxis against pre-eclampsia and intrauterine growth retardation, management of antiphospholipid syndrome (APS) and thromboprophylaxis in patients with valvular disease or mechanical prosthetic valves. Venous thromboembolism (VTE) continues to be the leading direct cause of maternal mortality in the United Kingdom [1] and VTE in pregnancy is an important cause of morbidity, not only during or immediately after pregnancy, but also in the long term [2]. Pregnancy and the puerperium are particular risk times for VTE, because of both the physiological changes in the coagulation factors causing a hypercoagulable state [3,4] and venous stasis [5,6]. All women should have an assessment of risk factors for VTE in early pregnancy.

There is now extensive experience in the use of low-molecular-weight heparins (LMWHs), which appear safe and effective for VTE prophylaxis and treatment in pregnancy. A clear understanding of the appropriate use of anticoagulants is essential for optimising management, in order to reduce acute morbidity and mortality and also to avoid the long-term complications of post-thrombotic syndrome. This chapter considers the use of LMWHs and other anticoagulants in the above situations in pregnancy.

Prescribing in Pregnancy, 4th edition. Edited by Peter Rubin and Margaret Ramsay,
 ISBN: 978-1-4051-4712-5.

Key points

Indications for anticoagulants in pregnancy

- Thromboprophylaxis and treatment of venous VTE
- Management of APS
- Prophylaxis against pre-eclampsia and intrauterine growth retardation
- Prophylaxis in patients with valvular disease or mechanical prosthetic valves

Heparins

Unfractionated heparin (UFH) is a naturally occurring mucopolysaccharide of varying chain length (5000 to >40,000 Da). However, the anticoagulant effect of UFH can be difficult to predict. After a standard dose of UFH, coagulation parameters must be monitored very closely to prevent over- or under-anticoagulation because of variable pharmacokinetics. UFH produces variable plasma levels depending on the degree of binding to proteins in the plasma and on the epithelium [7,8]. Close monitoring, usually with the activated partial thromboplastin time (aPTT), and dosage adjustment is required. In pregnancy, the aPTT response to heparin may be attenuated because of rise in some of the clotting factors (FVIII, fibrinogen) and proteins that bind heparin, therefore limiting the reliability of the test [9]. This means that the aPTT may not truly reflect the underlying anticoagulant status.

Recognised side effects include a 2% risk of symptomatic vertebral fracture secondary to osteoporosis, noted with prolonged usage, allergy and heparin-induced thrombocytopenia (HIT) [10]. HIT is an antibody-mediated reaction, with thrombocytopenia typically developing 5–10 days after commencing treatment, caused by antibodies against heparin–platelet complexes. There is a paradoxical risk of potentially life-threatening thrombus formation, and further exposure to any type of heparin is contraindicated. This, however, is a rare complication in pregnancy.

LMWHs consist of only short chains of polysaccharide. They are defined as heparin salts having an average molecular weight of less than 8000 Da. These are obtained by various methods of fractionation or depolymerisation of polymeric heparin. There are several LMWHs available in the UK, including enoxaparin, dalteparin and tinzaparin, which appear to have similar though not identical clinical effects. LMWHs have reliable pharmacokinetics and a long half-life, thus requiring less-frequent injections [11]. There is now considerable published experience in the use of LMWHs in pregnancy for thromboprophylaxis and treatment of VTE. There have been only five reports of osteoporotic fracture in the literature [12,13] and no cases of HIT occurring in pregnancy. Greer and Nelson-Piercy [14] performed a systematic review of all published studies up to the end of 2003. They included 64 studies reporting on 2777 pregnancies. The results demonstrated the safety and efficacy of LMWHs, with no maternal deaths. VTE occurred in 0.86% (95% confidence interval (CI), 0.55–1.28%) and arterial thrombosis associated with antiphospholipid syndrome in 0.5% (CI, 0.28–0.84%) of pregnancies. Significant bleeding occurred in 1.98% (95% CI, 1.34–2.57%), generally associated with primary obstetric causes, allergic skin reactions in 1.8% (95% CI, 1.34–2.37%), thrombocytopenia unrelated to heparin in 0.11% (95% CI, 0.02–0.2%), osteoporotic fracture in 0.04% (95% CI, <0.01–0.2%) and no cases of HIT.

Neither UFH nor the LMWHs cross the placenta, and there is no evidence of teratogenesis or risk of fetal haemorrhage. They are not excreted in breast milk and may be used safely during lactation.

Key points

Characteristics of heparins

- UFH requires regular monitoring with aPTT
- LMWHs are reliably absorbed and have a longer half-life
- UFH carries risk of allergy, HIT and osteoporosis; LMWHs have much lower risk
- Neither UFH nor LMWHs cross placenta; safe for breastfeeding

Other agents

Warfarin and other coumarins block activation of the vitamin K-dependent clotting factors. They cross the placenta and are both teratogenic and associated with a risk of fetal bleeding [15,16]. The embryopathy consists of nasal hypoplasia, stippled chondral calcification and scoliosis, and occurs principally between 6 and 12 weeks of gestation [17]. The risk may be dose-dependent, as doses greater than 5 mg/day have been associated with increased risk [18]. In addition, there is an association with risk of minor neurological dysfunction or low IQ [19]. Because of the increased risk of both fetal and maternal haemorrhage when coumarins are used in pregnancy, coumarins are stopped prior to delivery to reduce bleeding risk.

Danaparoid sodium (organon) is a LMWH, consisting of glycosaminoglycans. There is only a very small clinical risk of cross-reactivity with heparins and therefore in patients with allergic skin reactions or HIT, it may be used as an alternative. It does not cross the placenta and is not secreted into breast milk. There are anecdotal reports of its use in pregnancy [20,21].

Fondaparinux (arixtra) is a new antithrombotic agent, which is a synthetic pentasaccharide. This has been designated a category B drug in pregnancy from animal studies. However, there are very little data in human pregnancies. There are a few anecdotal case reports [22] and a small series of five cases [23]. There is evidence that this drug crosses the placenta [23], and animal studies indicate that it is secreted in milk [24]. Therefore, at present, it should only be used where alternative anticoagulation is unsuitable.

Lepirudin is a synthetic direct thrombin inhibitor. Its main use is in the setting of HIT. It is known to cross the placenta, and there are only a few case reports of its use in pregnancy in the mid- and third trimester [25,26].

Thrombolytic agents lyse clots by activating plasminogen, which in turn triggers fibrinolysis. The use of these agents will be limited to life-threatening thrombosis; bleeding is a major complication.

Aspirin is an anti-platelet agent rather than anticoagulant. It is not recommended for venous thromboprophylaxis [27]. It is shown to be safe in pregnancy in low dosage [28] and has a place in women with APS with recurrent miscarriage [29] and also in those rare cases of myeloproliferative syndrome where there is overproduction of platelets and/or red cells.

Key points

Other anticoagulant agents

- Coumarins cross the placenta, are teratogenic and can cause fetal bleeding
- Danaparoid sodium can be used for patients who have had HIT
- Fondaparinux is a new synthetic agent, with little experience of use in pregnancy
- Lepirudin is a direct thrombin inhibitor which crosses the placenta; it may be used in patients who have had HIT

Thromboprophylaxis of VTE

The decision to recommend thromboprophylaxis depends on identification of at-risk women early in pregnancy and a stratification of risk into those requiring antenatal and postpartum prophylaxis or postpartum prophylaxis only. In 2004, the Royal College of Obstetricians (RCOG) published guidelines on thromboprophylaxis in pregnancy, labour and the puerperium [30], listing risk factors and assessing levels of risk. Table 4.1 summarises the risk factors that need to be taken into consideration. At our institution, these guidelines have been adapted into an algorithm for planning thromboprophylaxis (Figure 4.1).

Antenatal prophylaxis

Previous personal history of VTE is associated with an overall increased recurrence risk of 3.5-fold. A prospective study demonstrated no antenatal recurrence in a group of women with prior VTE associated with a temporary risk factor and no thrombophilic defect but a 5.9% recurrence if the previous VTE was idiopathic or associated with a thrombophilia [31]. Previous pregnancy/pill-related events also have a higher recurrence rate as expected [31], and this appeared evenly spread through the three trimesters. Another study [32] showed a stepwise increase in incidence in each trimester, but still demonstrating a significant risk in the first trimester, indicating that prophylaxis should commence early in pregnancy. Women on long-term anticoagulation should change to LMWH before 6 weeks of gestation and treatment doses should be considered. In women with an identifiable thrombophilic marker but no personal thrombotic history, management will depend on the type and number of defects plus the assessment of other possible risk factors, in addition to review of family history.

Postnatal prophylaxis

All women judged to need antenatal prophylaxis will clearly also need peri- and postnatal thromboprophylaxis since VTE is significantly more common in the postpartum period than antenatally. Women judged at 'medium risk' (see Figure 4.1) will receive peri- and postpartum prophylaxis usually for a 6-week period. In addition, the RCOG guidelines recommend 5-day prophylaxis post-caesarean section for all women [33].

Table 4.1 Risk factors for VTE in pregnancy

Pre-existing	New onset or transient
Previous VTE	Surgical procedure in pregnancy or puerperium, e.g., evacuation of retained products of conception
Thrombophilias	Postpartum sterilisation
Congenital	Hyperemesis
Antithrombin deficiency	Dehydration
Protein C deficiency	Ovarian hyperstimulation syndrome
Protein S deficiency	Severe infection, e.g., pyelonephritis
Factor V Leiden	Immobility (>4-day bed rest)
Prothrombin gene variant	Pre-eclampsia
Acquired antiphospholipid syndrome	Excessive blood loss
Lupus anticoagulant	Long-haul travel
Anticardiolipin antibodies	Prolonged labour
Age over 35 yr	Midcavity instrumental delivery
Obesity (BMI $>$ 30 mg/m^2) pre-pregnancy or in early pregnancy	Immobility after delivery
Parity > 4	
Gross varicose veins	
Paraplegia	
Sickle cell disease	
Inflammatory disorders, e.g., inflammatory bowel disease	
Some medical disorders, e.g., nephritic syndrome, certain cardiac diseases	
Myeloproliferative disorders, e.g., essential thrombocythaemia	
Polycythaemia vera	

BMI, body mass index.

Standard management consists of once-daily use of a LMWH at a fixed dosage [34] (see Table 4.2). There is debate as to the need to monitor levels during pregnancy. Treatment should be omitted when in labour, to allow assessment and need for regional

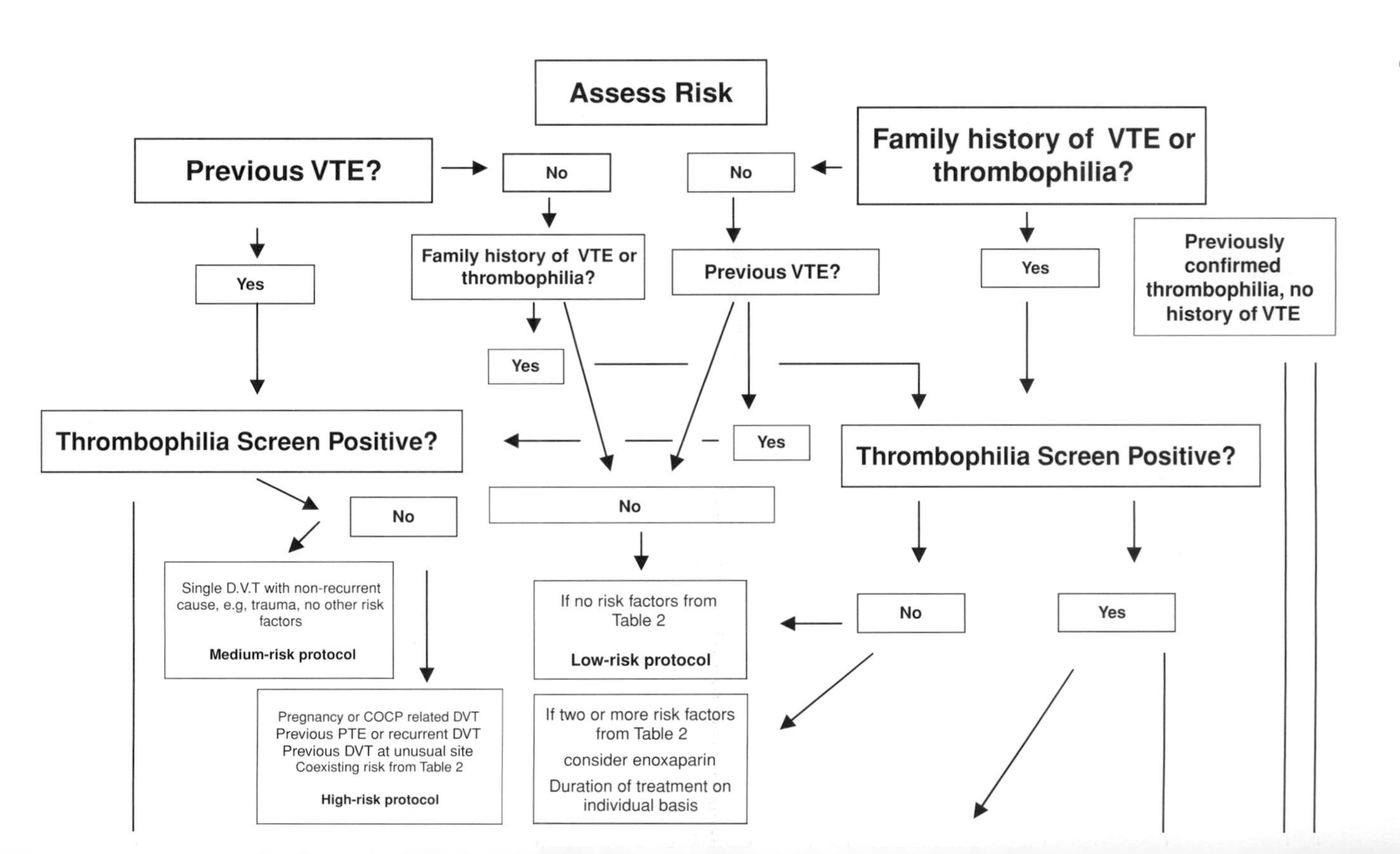
Assess Risk
Previous VTE?
No
No
Family history of VTE or thrombophilia?
Yes
Family history of VTE or thrombophilia?
Previous VTE?
Yes
Previously confirmed thrombophilia, no history of VTE
Yes
Yes
Thrombophilia Screen Positive?
Thrombophilia Screen Positive?
No
No
Single D.V.T with non-recurrent cause, e.g, trauma, no other risk factors
Medium-risk protocol
If no risk factors from Table 2
Low-risk protocol
No
Yes
Pregnancy or COCP related DVT
Previous PTE or recurrent DVT
Previous DVT at unusual site
Coexisting risk from Table 2
High-risk protocol
If two or more risk factors from Table 2
consider enoxaparin
Duration of treatment on individual basis

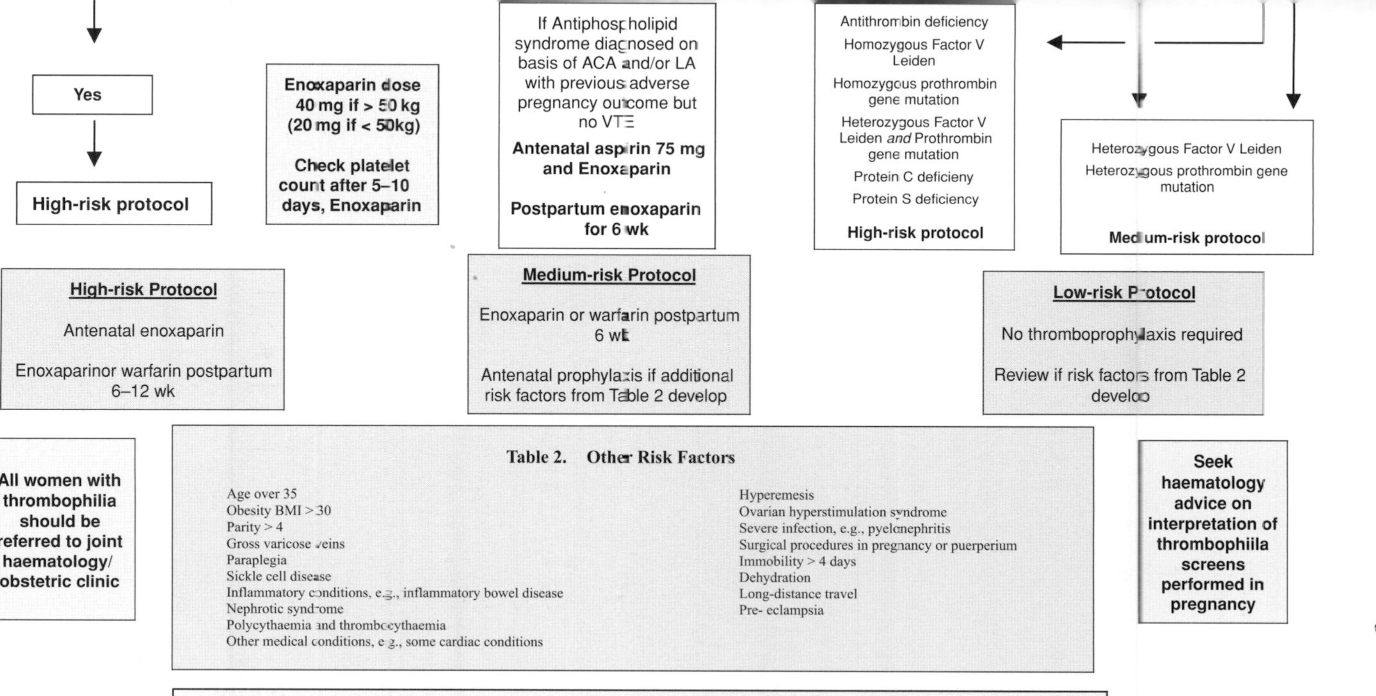

Figure 4.1 Planning thromboprophylaxis in pregnancy and the puerperium. DVT, deep vein thrombosis; COCP, combined oral contraceptive pill; ACA, anti-cardiolipin antibodies; LA, lupus anticoagulant; INR, international normalised ratio; LUSCS, lower uterine segment caesarean section; PTE, pulmonary thromboembolism; VTE, venous thromboembolism.
Reproduced with permission of the authors: J. Strong, J. Bingham, Nottingham University Hospitals, April 2004.

Table 4.2 Antenatal prophylactic and therapeutic doses of LMWH

Prophylaxis	Enoxaparin (100 units/mg)	Dalteparin	Tinzaparin
Normal body weight (50–90 kg)	40 mg daily	5000 units daily	4500 units daily
Body weight < 50 kg	20 mg daily	2500 units daily	3500 units daily
Body weight > 90 kg*	40 mg 12-hourly	5000 units 12-hourly	4500 units 12-hourly
Higher prophylactic dose	40 mg 12-hourly	5000 units 12-hourly	4500 units 12-hourly
Therapeutic dose	1 mg/kg 12-hourly	90 units/kg 12-hourly	90 units/kg 12-hourly

*BMI > 30 in early pregnancy.

anaesthesia. Regional anaesthesia should not be given within 10–12 hours of the prophylactic dose, because of the small risk of spinal haematoma [35,36]. A dose of LMWH may be given 3–4 hours after removal of the epidural/spinal catheter.

If LMWH is given while an epidural catheter is in situ, then this must not be removed for 10–12 hours after the injection [37]. Daily treatment is then resumed usually for 6 weeks. Conversion to warfarin is an alternative option postnatally, although there is a relative resistance to warfarinisation in the immediate postpartum period, due to the hypercoaguable state [38]. The inconvenience of regular INR checks plus the dual treatment of LMWH and warfarin until stabilised means that many women choose to remain on LMWH for the puerperium.

Key points

VTE prophylaxis

- Risk factors for VTE must be assessed early in pregnancy
- 2004 RCOG guidelines provide guidance on risk stratification
- Highest risk time for VTE is in the first 6 wk following delivery
- Antenatal VTEs occur in all three trimesters of pregnancy

Treatment of VTE

When VTE is suspected in pregnancy, anticoagulation should be commenced without delay, while awaiting confirmatory diagnostic tests. For the majority of patients, the treatment will be with LMWH in twice-daily weight-related dosage [39] (which differs from the regimen used outwith pregnancy (see Table 4.2.) There is good evidence in non-pregnant patients of the equivalence in safety and efficacy of LMWH to UFH.

LMWHs have a lower risk of bleeding complications and mortality rate in non-pregnant patients compared to UFH [40]. Pregnancy guidelines have been produced based on this evidence in non-pregnant patients and on the body of information accumulated from use in pregnancy of both agents (RCOG, ACCP [27, 39]).

These state that two approaches are acceptable:

1 Initial UFH followed by at least 3-month subcutaneous LMWH in therapeutic doses or dose-adjusted subcutaneous UFH.
2 Therapeutic dose LMWH or adjusted dose UFH given subcutaneously, used for both acute and long-term treatment.

Dose adjustments of UFH are dependent on careful monitoring of the aPTT. In addition to the apparent heparin resistance due to the increase of various clotting factors during pregnancy, audits show this to be poorly performed. However, in a situation where a VTE has occurred near to term and close attention is paid to careful monitoring, the short half-life of intravenous UFH (1–2 h) is advantageous, enabling tight control of anticoagulation during labour. Where risk is considered very high, an inferior vena cava filter may be inserted to further reduce risk of embolism during labour. A relatively new type of temporary filter is now available, which may be left in situ for a number of months, rather than the previous maximum of 7–10 days, which further assists management of this high-risk period. When UFH is used short- or long-term, platelet counts must be checked at 1 and 2 weeks and then monthly to exclude HIT. Immediate discontinuation of heparin and substitution with danaparoid should be instituted. Treatment with LMWHs is monitored by an anti-Xa assay, 3–4 hours after a morning dose. Twice-daily treatment is preferable in pregnancy [41,42] as the half-life of LMWHs is reduced due to increased renal clearance [43]. It is not necessary to check platelet counts in women treated with LMWHs unless previously exposed to UFH [44].

Guidelines recommend a duration of 6 months at treatment doses. Where a VTE has occurred early in pregnancy, the dose may be reduce to prophylactic levels after this time, provided there are no additional risk factors. Following delivery, treatment should be continued for at least 6 weeks. Dosage is often reduced around the time of expected delivery and the woman is instructed to omit the heparin when in labour.

Epidural or spinal anaesthesia cannot be given for at least 24 hours after a treatment dose of LMWH and 10–12 hours after a prophylactic dose. Timing of removal of the epidural catheter is as above.

Key points

Treatment of VTE

- If VTE is suspected, treatment must be started immediately, while awaiting tests
- Treatment doses and frequencies differ from those in non-pregnant cases
- Epidural or spinal anaesthesia is contraindicated if within 24 h of a full treatment dose

Management of APS

Low-titre antiphospholipid antibodies (aPL) are common in pregnancy and are not significant; the APS is a condition defined by clinical and strict laboratory criteria [45].

These are summarised below:

Clinical features: pregnancy morbidity

a One fetal death at/after 10 weeks with normal fetal morphology

b Premature birth before 34 weeks of gestation due to:
- severe pre-eclampsia/eclampsia
- recognised features of placental insufficiency, e.g.:
  - abnormal fetal surveillance tests
  - abnormal umbilical artery Doppler signals

– oligohydramnios
– birth weight < 10th centile for age

c Three or more unexplained miscarriages (<10 wk)

Clinical features: thrombotic events

a Venous or arterial thrombosis – cerebral vascular system, coronary arteries, pulmonary emboli, hepatic/renal veins

b Small vessel thrombotic events

Laboratory features

Demonstration of one or more aPL present on two occasions at least 12 weeks apart:

a anticardiolipin antibodies of medium or high titre
b anti-beta 2 glycoprotein 1 antibodies
c lupus anticoagulant

Patients with previous thrombotic events and APS should have received pre-pregnancy counselling. These patients may be on long-term anticoagulation and need counselling on the thrombotic and miscarriage risks in pregnancy and specific discussion on changing from warfarin to heparin. The aims in management of the pregnancy are to maximise chance of successful fetal outcome and to prevent thrombosis and other clinical problems in the mother.

With regards to pregnancy outcome, there have been several trials. Although APS is an immune disorder, there is no evidence that steroids improve live birth rate, and additionally it may cause maternal and fetal morbidity [46,47]. One randomised, controlled trial (RCT) in women with recurrent miscarriage and aPLs demonstrated a live birth rate of 40% when treated with aspirin alone, and an improvement to 70% when a combination of low-dose aspirin and LMWH was used [48]. Another RCT reported high success rate with aspirin alone and no significant benefit in live birth rate with the addition of heparin [29]. However, this trial has been criticised for inclusion of women with low titres of aPL and randomisation at up to 12 weeks of gestation, by which time most of aPL-related pregnancy losses would have already occurred. A meta-analysis of three trials examining the role of aspirin alone compared with placebo or supportive care found no significant benefit [49]. Finally, a meta-analysis of two controlled trials concluded that in women with recurrent miscarriage and aPL, treatment with low-dose heparin plus low-dose aspirin significantly reduced the pregnancy losses by 54% when compared with aspirin alone [49]. Pregnancies associated with aPL treated with aspirin and heparin remain at high risk of complications during all three trimesters [48,50,51].

Key points

APS

- Low-titre antibodies are common in pregnancy and are not significant
- Pregnancy in women with APS remains high risk for complications
- Treatment with low-dose aspirin and LMWH significantly improves outcome

Prevention of pregnancy complications associated with thrombophilias

Several studies suggested a link between hereditary and acquired thrombophilic status and adverse pregnancy outcomes, including fetal loss in all three trimesters, pre-eclampsia and intrauterine growth restriction. Most studies are limited by poor methodology or focus on only one pregnancy complication [52–57]. However, more recently, comprehensive meta-analyses confirm that women with thrombophilia are at increased risk of pregnancy complications [58–60]; they also identify the fact that although the relative risk is increased, the absolute risk remains low and therefore there is no case for universal screening.

One to three per cent of women have recurrent pregnancy losses (RPL) of three or more miscarriages [61]. Small studies suggest thromboprophylaxis with LMWH significantly improves gestational outcome [52,53,62,63]. More recently, a large, prospective, case-controlled trial [64] has been conducted in women with one fetal loss after 10 weeks and a thrombophilic disorder. LMWH (enoxaparin, 40 mg o.d.) was compared with low-dose aspirin (100 mg o.d.), both commencing from the eighth week. This study demonstrated dramatic superiority of enoxaparin over aspirin in live-birth outcome (OR, 15.5; 95% CI, 7–34, $p < 0.001$) and also in subgroup analysis of individual thrombophilias (including protein C deficiency, protein S deficiency and Factor V Leiden). The birth weight was higher in the enoxaparin group and small-for-dates babies were seen more frequently in the aspirin-treated group. There may be a place to consider LMWH in women with RPL, regardless of the presence or absence of a thrombophilic marker [65].

There are currently trials in progress addressing this issue. The addition of low-dose aspirin to the LMWH regime is controversial. Although this combination appears effective in the setting of APS, the underlying pathophysiology here may not be comparable and studies are needed in this area to optimise treatment for this group of women. It is a recognised problem, however, that recruiting to randomised studies is problematic in women who have suffered multiple miscarriages.

Key points

Pregnancy complications and thrombophilia

- Studies show improved outcome for RPL with LMWHs
- Future studies needed to clarify place for LMWHs in RPL without thrombophilia
- Randomised studies in this group of women are difficult to perform

Management of anticoagulant therapy in patients with prosthetic heart valves

The management of pregnant women with prosthetic valves poses a significant challenge, because of the apparent thrombotic risk to the mother of heparin preparations versus the risks to the baby of warfarin (teratogenesis, neurodevelopmental problems and bleeding). A systematic review carried out by Chan et al. [17] analysed outcomes for mother and fetus in the three most commonly used regimes.

These were:

1 use of warfarin throughout the pregnancy
2 replacing warfarin with UFH for weeks 6–12 gestation
3 UFH use throughout.

Heparin was used at term in all the groups to avoid delivery with an anticoagulated fetus. The use of warfarin throughout was associated with the lowest risk of thromboembolic problems (3.9%) but also with warfarin embryopathy in 6.4% of live births. Replacing warfarin with UFH in the first trimester abolished incidence of embryopathy but was associated with an increased incidence of valve thrombosis (9.2%). Use of UFH throughout the pregnancy had an alarming rate of valve thrombosis, 60% when used at low dose and 25% with adjusted doses. The authors comment on the limitations of this study: The patients were a heterogeneous group in terms of type and site of valve (two-thirds had a mitral valve prosthesis and 50% had cage and ball valves, both features of higher risk), presence of arrhythmias, type of study and accuracy of reporting. Numbers in the studies reviewed were generally small. It is difficult to extrapolate this data to the less thrombogenic newer valves and to use of LMWHs. There a number of case studies reporting valve thrombosis and stoke associated with LMWHs [66–70]. The use of LMWHs in pregnant women with heart valves has been systematically reviewed by Oran et al. [71]. Sixty-seven pregnancies in women with prosthetic valves treated with various doses of LMWH were assessed. Valve thrombosis occurred in 7 cases (10.4%). The total thromboembolic incidence was 13.4% (9/67), and a mortality rate was of 1.49%. In 8 of the 9 instances of thrombotic event, the patient had received a fixed rather than adjusted dose of LMWH, and in 2 cases this was a fixed low dosage. Anti-Xa levels were monitored in 42 pregnancies, and in this group there was only one thromboembolic complication. There was a 90% live-birth rate and no congenital abnormalities.

There is still a relative dearth of data to guide management of these women, and several approaches are acceptable. If LMWHs are employed, close monitoring of the anti-Xa level is essential, maintaining high levels of 1.0–1.2, and a similar tight control of adjusted-dose UFH is necessary. Use of warfarin between 13 and 36 weeks is commonly employed. Aspirin in low dose may be added to heparin use [72]. Studies designed to clarify the difficult issues surrounding the management of these patients are necessary.

Key points

Anticoagulation and mechanical heart valves

- Management continues to be a challenge with all treatments problematic
- Inadequate up-to-date information to guide best treatment choice
- Warfarin appears to be best in thrombosis prevention, but with risk of fetal problems
- Heparins appear to have higher risk of serious valve thrombosis

Conclusion

Anticoagulants are used for an increasing number of indications in pregnancy. The management and prophylaxis of VTEs in pregnancy has been much simplified by the introduction of LMWHs. Awareness of the importance of accurate and early risk assessments in pregnancy has led to a growing number of women receiving antenatal and postpartum prophylaxis for high-risk cases or postpartum prophylaxis alone for the medium-risk patients. While there are a variety of risk-scoring systems, similar prophylactic strategies are emerging and hopefully will be reflected in further reduction in morbidity and mortality from VTE in pregnancy. There is relatively clear guidance in the case of APS, but further studies are required in the areas of prevention of pregnancy complications and for the management of women with metallic valves.

References

1 Drife J for CEMACH (Confidential Enquiry into Maternal and Child Health). Thrombosis and thrombo-embolism. In: *Why Mothers Die 2000–2002*. London: RCOG Press; 2004, Chapter 2.

2 McColl MD, Ellison J, Greer IA, Tait RC, Walker ID. Prevalence of the post-thrombotic syndrome in young women with previous venous thromboembolism, *Br J Haematol* 2000 **108**(2):272–4.

3 Clarke P, Brennand J, Conkie JA, McCall F, Greer IA, Walker ID. Activated protein C sensitivity, protein C, protein S and coagulation in normal pregnancy. *Thromb Haemost* 1998;**79**:1166–70.

4 Greer IA. Haemostasis and thrombosis in pregnancy. In: Bloom AL, Forbes CD, Thomas DP, Tuddenham EGD (eds.), *Haemostasis and Thrombosis*. Churchill Livingstone: Edinburgh; 1994:987–1015.

5 Macklon NS, Greer IA. The deep leg venous system in the puerperium. An ultrasound study. *Br J Obstet Gynaecol* 1997;**104**:198–200.

6 Lindhagen A, Bergqvist A, Bergqvist D, Hallbook T. Late venous function in the leg after deep venous thrombosis occurring in relation to pregnancy. *Br J Obstet Gynaecol* 1996;**93**:348–52.

7 Glimelius B, Busch C, Hook M. Binding of heparin on the surface of cultured endothelial cells. *Thromb Res* 1978;**12**:73–82.

8 Young E, Prins M, Levine MN, Hirsch J. Heparin binding to plasma proteins, an important mechanism for heparin resistance. *Thromb Haemost* 1992;**79**:1–17.

9 Hyers TM, Hull RD, Weg JG. Antithrombotic therapy for venous thrombo-embolic disease. *Chest* 1995;**108**:335s–51s.

10 Nelson-Piercy C. Hazards of heparin: allergy, heparin-induced thrombocytopenia and osteoporosis. In: Greer IA (ed.), *Bailliere's Clinical Obstetrics and Gynaecology – Thromboembolic Disease in Obstetrics and Gynaecology.* London: Bailliere Tindall; 1997:489–509.
11 Weitz JL. Low molecular weight heparins. *N Engl J Med* 1997;**337**:688–98.
12 Hunt BJ, Doughty H, Majurnder G, et al. Thromboprophylaxis with low molecular weight heparin (Fragmin) in high risk pregnancies. *Thromb Haemost* 1997;**77**:39–43.
13 Byrd LM, Johnston TA, Shiach C, Hay C. Osteopenic fractures and low molecular weight heparin in pregnancy. *J Obstet Gynaecol* 2004; **2451**:1113–7.
14 Greer IA, Nelson-Piercy C. Low-molecular weight heparins for thromboprophylaxis and treatment of venous thromboembolism in pregnancy: a systemic review of safety and efficacy. *Blood* 2005;**106**(2): 401–7.
15 Bates SM, Ginsberg JS. Anticoagulants in pregnancy: fetal defects. In: Greer IA (ed.), *Bailliere's Clinical Obstetrics and Gynaecology*. London: Bailliere Tindall; 1997:479–88.
16 Bates S, Greer IA, Ginsberg J, Hirsh J. Use of antithrombotic agents during pregnancy. *Chest* 2004;**126**(Suppl 3):627s–44s.
17 Chan WS, Anand S, Ginsberg JS. Anticoagulation of pregnant women with mechanical heart valves. *Arch Intern Med* 2000;**160**:191–6.
18 Vitale N, De Feo M, De Santo LS, Pollice A, Tedesco N, Cotrufo M. Dose-dependent fetal complications of warfarin in pregnant women with mechanical heart valves. *J Am Coll Cardiol* 1999;**33**:1637–41.
19 Wesseling J, van Driel D, Heymans HAS, et al. Coumarins during pregnancy: long-term effects on growth and development of school-age children. *Thromb Haemost* 2001;**85**(4):577–755.
20 Myers B, Westby J, Strong J. Prophylactic use of danaparoid in high-risk pregnancy with heparin-induced thrombocytopenia positive skin reaction. *Blood Coagul Fibrinolysis* 2003;**14**:485–7.
21 Schindlewolf M, Mosch G, Bauersachs RM, Lindhoff-Last E. Safe anticoagulation with danaparoid in pregnancy and lactation. *Thromb Haemost* 2004;**92**(1):211.
22 Wijesiriwardana A, Lees DA, Lush C. Fondaparinux as anticoagulant in a pregnant woman with heparin allergy. *Blood Coagul* 2006;**17**(2):147–9.
23 Dempfle CE. Minor transplacental passage of fondaparinux in vivo. *N Engl J Med* 2004;**350**:1914–5.
24 Fondaparinux sodium package insert. West Orange, NJ: Organon/ Sanofi-Synthelabo LLC, January 2002.
25 Harenberg J, Jorg I, Bayerl C, Fiehn C. Treatment of a woman with lupus pernio, thrombosis and cutaneous intolerance to heparins using lepirudin during pregnancy. *Lupus* 2005;**14**(5):411–2.

26 Huhle G, Geberth M, Hoffman U, Heene DL, Harenberg J. Management of heparin-associated thrombocytopenia in pregnancy with subcutaneous r-hirudin. *Gynaecol Obstet Invest* 2000;**49**:67–9.
27 Geerts WH, Pineo GF, Heit JA, et al. Prevention of venous thromboembolism. ACCP guidelines. *Chest* 2004;**126**:343S.
28 CLASP (Collaborative Low-dose Aspirin Study in Pregnancy) Collaborative Group. CLASP: a randomised trial of low-dose aspirin for the prevention and treatment of pre-eclampsia among 9364 pregnant women. *Lancet* 1994;**343**:619–29.
29 Farquharson RG, Quenby S, Greaves M. Antiphosholipid syndrome in pregnancy: a randomised, controlled trial of treatment. *Obstet Gynaecol* 2002;**100**:408–13.
30 Royal College of Obstetricians and Gynaecologists. *Thromboprophylaxis During Pregnancy, Labour and After Vaginal Delivery.* Guideline Number 37. London: RCOG Press; 2004.
31 Pabinger I, Grafenhofer H, Kyrle PA, et al. Risk of pregnancy-associated recurrent venous thromboembolism in women with a history of venous thrombosis. *J Thromb Haemost* 2005;**3**(5):949–54.
32 Voke J, Hunt BJ, Keidan J, Pavord S, Spencer N,on behalf of the British Society for Haematology Obstetric Haematology Group. The management of antenatal venous thromboembolism in the UK and Ireland: a prospective multicentre survey. *Br J* Haematol, submitted.
33 Royal College of Obstetricians and Gynaecologists. *Report of the RCOG Working Party on Prophylaxis Against Thromboembolism in Gynaecology and Obstetrics*. London: RCOG Press; 1995.
34 Greer IA, Hunt BJ. Low molecular weight heparin in pregnancy: current issues. *Br J Haematol* 2005;**128**:593–601.
35 Baron EM, Burke JA, Akhtar N, Young WV. Spinal epidural haematoma associated with tissue plasminogen activator treatment of acute myocardial infarction. *Cathet Cardiovasc Intervent* 1999;**48**:390–6.
36 Shaieb MD, Watson BN, Atkinson RE. Bleeding complications with enoxaparin for deep venous thrombosis prophylaxis. *J Arthroplasty* 1999;**14**:432–8.
37 American Society of Regional Anesthesia and Pain Medicine. Second consensus statement, 2002. Available at: http://www.asra.com.
38 British Society for Haematology. Guidelines on oral anticoagulation: third edition. *Br J Haematol* 1998;**101**:374–87.
39 Thompson AJ, Greer IA. Royal College of Obstetricians and Gynaecologists. *Thromboembolic Disease in Pregnancy and the Puerperium: Acute Management*. Guideline Number 28. London: RCOG Press; 2001.
40 Hull RD, Raskob GE, Pineo GF, et al. Subcutaneous low-molecular-weight heparin compared with continuous intravenous heparin in the treatment of proximal-vein thrombosis. *N Engl J Med* 1992;**326**:975–82.

41 Rodie VA, Thompson AJ, Stewart FM, Quinn AJ, Walker ID, Greer IA. Low molecular weight heparin, for the treatment of venous thromboembolism in pregnancy: a case series. *BJOG* 2002; **109**:1020–4.
42 Merli G, Spiro TE, Olsson CG, et al. Subcutaneous enoxaparin once or twice daily compared with intravenous unfractionated heparin for treatment of venous thromboembolic disease. *Ann Intern Med* 2001;**134**:192–202.
43 Casele HL, Laifer SA, Woelkers DA, Venkataramanan R. Changes in pharmacokinetics of the low molecular molecular heparin enoxaparin during pregnancy. *Am J Obstet Gynaecol* 1999;**181**:1113–7.
44 Warkentin TE, Greinacher A. Heparin-induced thrombocytopenia: recognition, treatment and prevention. 7th ACCP conference on antithrombotic and thrombolytic therapy. *Chest* 2004;**126**(Suppl 3):311S–37S.
45 Miyakis S, Lockshin MD, Atsumi T, et al. International consensus statement on an update of the classification criteria for definite antiphospholipid syndrome (APS). *J Thromb Haemost* 2006;**4**(2): 295–306.
46 Cowchock FS, Reece EA, Balaban D, Branch DW, Plouffe L. Repeated fetal losses associated with antiphospholipid antibodies: a collaborative randomised trial comparing prednisolone with low-dose heparin treatment. *Am J Obstet Gynaecol* 1992;**166**:1318–23.
47 Silver RK, MacGregor SN, Sholl JS, Hobart JM, Neerhof MG, Ragin A. Comparative trial of prednisolone plus aspirin versus aspirin alone in the treatment of anticardiolipin antibody-positive obstetric patients. *Am J Obstet Gynaecol* 1993;**169**:1411–7.
48 Rai RS, Cohen H, Dave M, Regan L. Randomised controlled trial of aspirin and aspirin plus heparin in pregnant women with recurrent miscarriage associated with phospholipid antibodies (or antiphospholipid antibodies). *Br Med J* 1997;**314**:253–7.
49 Empson M, Lassere M, Craig JC, Scott JR. Recurrent pregnancy loss with antiphospholipid antibody: a systemic review of therapeutic trials. *Obstet Gynaecol* 2002;**99**:135–44.
50 Backos M, Rai R, Baxter N, Chilcott IT, Cohen H, Regan L. Pregnancy complications in women with recurrent miscarriage associated with antiphospholipid antibodies treated with low-dose aspirin and heparin. *Br J Obstet Gynaecol* 1999;**106**:102–7.
51 Branch DW, Silver RM, Blackwell JL, Reading JC, Scott JR. Outcome of treated pregnancies in women with antiphospholipid syndrome: an update of the Utah experience. *Obstet Gynaecol* 1992;**80**: 614–20.
52 Preston FE, Rosendaal FR, Walker ID, et al. Increased fetal loss in women with hereditable thrombophilia. *Lancet* 1996;**348**: 913–6.
53 Brenner B. Clinical management of thrombophilia-related placental vascular complication. *Blood* 2004;**103**:4003–9.

54 Sanson BJ, Friederich PW, Simioni P. The risk of abortion and still-birth in anti-thrombin, protein C, and protein S deficient women. *Thromb Haemost* 1996;**75**:387–8.

55 Vossen CY, Preston FE, Conard J, et al. Hereditary thrombophilia and fetal loss: a prospective follow-up study. *J Thromb Haemost* 2004;**2**:592–6.

56 Gris JC, Quere L, Monperyroux F, et al. Case-control study of the frequency of thrombophilic disorders in couples with late fetal loss and no thrombotic antecedant – the Nimes Obstetricians and Haematologists study 5 (NOHA5). *Thromb Haemost* 1999; **81**:891–9.

57 Kupferminc MJ, Eldor A, Steinman N, et al. Increased frequency of genetic thrombophilia in women with complications of pregnancy. *N Engl J Med* 1999;**340**:50–2.

58 Rey E, Kahn SR, David M, Shrier I. Thrombophilic disorders and fetal loss: a meta-analysis. *Lancet* 2003;**361**:901–8.

59 Robertson L, Wu O, Langhorne P, et al. Thrombophilia and pregnancy: a systemic review. *Br J Haematol* 2005;**132**:171–96.

60 Kovalevsky G, Gracia CR, Berlin JA, Sammel MD, Barnhart KT. Evaluation of the association between hereditary thrombophilias and recurrent pregnancy loss. *Arch Intern Med* 2004;**164**:558–63.

61 Stirrat GM. Recurrent miscarriage. *Lancet* 1990;**336**:673–5.

62 Carp H, Dolitzky M, Inbal A. Thromboprophylaxis improves the live birth rate in women with consecutive recurrent miscarriages and hereditary thrombophilia. *J Thromb Haemost* 2003;**1**:433–8.

63 Brenner B, Hoffman R, Blumenfeld Z, Weiner Z, Younis J. Gestational outcome in thrombophilic women with recurrent pregnancy loss treated by enoxaparin. *Thromb Haemost* 2000;**83**:693–7.

64 Gris JC, Mercier E, Quere I, et al. Low-molecular weight heparin versus low dose aspirin in women with one fetal loss and a constitutional thrombophilic disorder. *Blood* 2004;**103**(10):3695–9.

65 Greer IA. Procoagulant microparticles: new insights and opportunities in pregnancy loss? *Thromb Haemost* 2001;**85**:3–4.

66 Idir M, Madonna F, Roudaut R. Collapse and massive pulmonary oedema secondary to thrombosis of a mitral mechanical valve prosthesis during low-molecular weight heparin therapy. *J Heart Valve Dis* 1999;**8**: 303–4.

67 Berndt N, Khan I, Gallo R. A complication in anticoagulation using low-molecular weight heparin in a patient with mechanical valve prosthesis. A case report. *J Heart Valve Dis* 2000;**9**:844–6.

68 Lev-Ran O, Kramer A, Gurevitch J, Shapira I, Mohr R. Low molecular weight heparin for prosthetic heart valves: treatment failure. *Ann Thorac Surg* 2000;**69**:264–5.

69 Roberts N, Ross D, Flint SK, Arya R, Blott M. Thromboembolism in pregnant women with mechanical prosthetic heart valves anticoagulated with low molecular weight heparin. *BJOG* 2001;**108**:327–9.

70 Mahesh B, Evans S, Bryan AJ. Failure of low molecular weight heparin in the prevention of prosthetic mitral valve thrombosis during pregnancy: case report and review of the options for anticoagulation. *J Heart Valve Dis* 2002;**11**:745–50.
71 Oran B, Lee-Paritz A, Ansell J. Low molecular weight heparin for the prophylaxis of thromboembolism in women with prosthetic mechanical heart valves during pregnancy. *Thromb Haemost* 2004;**94**:747–51.
72 Turpie AG, Gent M, Laupacis A, et al. Comparison of aspirin with placebo in patients treated with warfarin after heart valve replacement. *N Engl J Med* 1993;**329**:524–9.

CHAPTER 5
Treatment of cardiovascular diseases

Asma Khalil, Pat O'Brien

Introduction

Women may develop cardiovascular disease for the first time in pregnancy; this may be either pregnancy-related (such as pre-eclampsia) or due to the unmasking of a previously undiagnosed condition, such as mitral stenosis. Women with pre-existing cardiovascular disease will need careful management in pregnancy; the normal physiological changes associated with the pregnant state (and persisting for a variable period after birth) place extra demand on the cardiovascular system. Ideally, care should be delivered in a specialised centre by a multidisciplinary team including an obstetrician, cardiologist, haematologist and anaesthetist, all with expertise in this area.

Only 4% of developmental disorders are caused by chemical and physical agents, of which only a small proportion are due to medicinal products [1]. However, the list of known embryo/fetotoxic drugs includes several used in cardiac patients, including angiotensin-converting enzyme inhibitors (ACE inhibitors), phenytoin and warfarin. When prescribing a new drug, particularly for long-term medication, for a woman of reproductive age, the possibility of pregnancy should be raised, appropriate contraception arranged and, if pregnancy is planned, treatment adjusted accordingly.

The commonest cardiovascular conditions faced by the clinician are hypertensive disorders and arrhythmias. However, the demographics of the pregnant population are changing: the average age

Prescribing in Pregnancy, 4th edition. Edited by Peter Rubin and Margaret Ramsay,
 ISBN: 978-1-4051-4712-5.

is rising, and so age-related conditions, such as ischaemic heart disease, are being encountered more commonly in pregnancy. In addition, a cohort of women who themselves had congenital heart disease is now becoming pregnant. Until recently, such women either did not survive into the reproductive years or were advised to avoid pregnancy. Now for the first time, however, these women are becoming pregnant; they often have complex cardiac circulations and may be taking a range of cardiovascular drugs, including anticoagulants.

Antihypertensives

The most commonly used antihypertensives in pregnancy are α-methyldopa, nifedipine, labetalol and hydralazine. It is important to remember that pre-eclampsia is a multisystem endothelial disorder and that antihypertensive treatment, while helping to control maternal hypertension, does little to alter the course of the underlying pathology.

Methyldopa – This is regarded as safe throughout pregnancy [2]. Although it crosses the placenta, there have been no reports of adverse fetal effects [3,4], and long-term paediatric follow-up over 7 years found no evidence of long-term abnormalities in children of mothers treated in pregnancy [5].

Methyldopa is a central nervous depressant and may cause maternal drowsiness, depression and postural hypotension. It has a similar effect on the fetus, which results in reduced fetal heart rate variability on the cardiotocograph. Despite this, methyldopa remains the first-line drug for essential hypertension in the months before conception and for antihypertensive treatment started during pregnancy. Because of the association with depression, however, it is usually replaced postnatally by an alternative such as a β-blocker.

Calcium channel antagonists – The most common one in pregnancy is nifedipine, but the use of nicardipine, nitrendipine and isradipine has also been described. Several large studies have shown that calcium channel blockers in the second and third trimesters (when they are most often used) are effective antihypertensives and have no significant adverse effects [6–11]. A prospective cohort study of patients contacting teratogen information services in Canada showed no increase in fetal malformations with exposure to calcium antagonists in the first trimester [12].

Some case reports raised concerns about the possible synergistic effect of nifedipine and magnesium sulphate (a common combination in women with pre-eclampsia), leading to serious hypotensive reactions [13]. However, the large MAGPIE Trial found no evidence of such synergy and indeed found that magnesium sulphate did not seem to have any antihypertensive effect [14].

Hydralazine – This is a vasodilator which, in pregnancy, is usually given parenterally in the acute management of hypertension (see below).

β-Adrenergic receptor blockers (β-blockers) – This class includes a long list of drugs including atenolol, bisoprolol, esmolol, labetalol, metoprolol, oxprenolol, pindolol, propranolol, sotalol and timolol. The most commonly used in pregnancy are labetalol and atenolol. They are most commonly used in pregnancy as antihypertensives or antiarrhythmics, but also have less common uses such as in migraine or Marfan syndrome. Many have both β-1 and β-2 activity; labetalol is primarily a non-selective β-blocker with some weak α-blocking activity. All β-blockers cross the placenta. From the evidence available to date, β-blockers do not seem to be teratogenic following exposure in the first trimester [15].

Some studies have found an increased risk of intrauterine growth restriction (IUGR), particularly with longer term treatment with higher doses [16,17]. However, the underlying maternal disease may well explain this effect, and other controlled studies have found no difference in the rates of IUGR between the exposed and non-exposed groups [15,18]. A Cochrane review [19] of 12 trials of β-blockers versus placebo/no treatment for mild to moderate hypertension suggested that IUGR was more common with β-blockers (relative risk, 1.36; 95% confidence interval (CI), 1.02–1.82). However, when the Butters' trial [17] (which used large doses from an early gestation) was excluded, the relative risk fell to 1.30 and failed to achieve statistical significance (95% CI, 0.97–1.74). A more recent meta-analysis of various antihypertensives for mild to moderate hypertension in pregnancy found that the treatment-induced fall in mean arterial pressure was proportional to the increased risk of IUGR [20]. The authors concluded that this effect was not specific to β-blockers, but that hypertension over-treated with *any* antihypertensive could impair placental perfusion and lead to IUGR. IUGR could theoretically also be mediated through the lowering of blood sugar by β-receptor blockade.

However, postnatal growth and development does not seem to be affected [21].

In summary, the risk of IUGR associated with the use of β-blockers in pregnancy seems small, particularly when large doses are avoided, and their use is confined to the third trimester. When used, hypertension should not be over-treated and fetal growth should be monitored with serial growth scans. If β-blockers are used up to the time of delivery, there is a theoretical risk of neonatal bradycardia, hypotension and hypoglycaemia due to the β-blocking effect [22]. However, in practice such adverse effects seem rare.

ACE inhibitors – This class of drugs includes *captopril, enalapril, lisinopril, ramipril* and others. ACE inhibitors inhibit the conversion of angiotensin I to angiotensin II. Their use outside pregnancy has become more widespread in recent years, but most available data on their use in pregnancy refer to captopril and enalapril. However, it is likely that the other drugs in this class have similar fetal and neonatal effects.

Recently published data show that the use of ACE inhibitors in the first trimester is associated with an increased risk of major congenital abnormalities, especially those of the cardiovascular or central nervous system (risk ratio, 2.71; 95% CIs, 1.72–4.27) [23]. Detailed ultrasound examination of fetal structures, including careful cardiac assessment should be offered at 18–22 weeks of gestation. Any woman discovering that she is pregnant whilst taking an ACE inhibitor should be changed to another antihypertensive agent, if possible. Inadvertent exposure to ACE inhibitors in the first trimester is not considered an indication for termination of pregnancy or invasive diagnostic procedures.

Exposure in the second and third trimesters can cause marked fetal hypotension and decreased (fetal) renal blood flow, occasionally even leading to fetal renal failure in utero. Severe oligohydramnios may result in pulmonary hypoplasia, limb contractures and craniofacial deformities. IUGR and preterm delivery have been reported. These adverse effects persist in the neonate, with poor renal perfusion and glomerular filtration rate; there may be significant hypotension and renal failure severe enough to cause neonatal death. Where ACE inhibitors must be continued, amniotic fluid volume and fetal growth should be monitored carefully. Blood pressure and renal function should be monitored closely in the neonate [24].

Angiotensin II inhibitors – These include *losartan* and *valsartan*. These are specific angiotensin II receptor antagonists and consequently have properties similar to ACE Inhibitors. These are relatively recent drugs and data in pregnancy are still scanty, but it seems likely that they will cause the same toxic fetal effects observed with ACE inhibitors in the second and third trimesters [25]. Consequently these drugs are not recommended in pregnancy unless all other treatment avenues have been explored.

Prazosin – This is an α-adrenoreceptor blocker which has occasionally been used in pregnancy as a second-line antihypertensive treatment, usually in combination with a β-blocker [26]. It appears safe, but precautions should be taken against first-dose hypotension.

Hypertensive emergencies

The definitive treatment for uncontrolled hypertension and pre-eclampsia is delivery. Nevertheless, blood pressure must be controlled in labour or before anaesthesia. The most commonly used agents are intravenous (i.v.) hydralazine or labetalol, or oral nifedipine.

When *hydralazine* or *labetalol* are given i.v., there is a significant risk of a precipitate fall in blood pressure, which may lead to impaired placental perfusion and fetal heart rate abnormalities. Consequently, *slow* i.v. administration is mandatory [27].

When *nifedipine* is used in this situation, care must also be exercised to avoid too rapid a fall in blood pressure. For this reason, the sublingual route should be avoided, oral (and even the slow-release formulation) is preferable.

Magnesium sulphate is the drug of choice for the *primary* prevention of seizures in women with severe pre-eclampsia [14], and for the prevention of *recurrent* seizures in eclampsia [28]. As mentioned above, there had been concerns about the possible synergistic effect of calcium channel antagonists and magnesium on blood pressure, but this has largely been discounted by the MAGPIE Trial [14].

Prevention of pre-eclampsia

Aspirin – It has long been known that platelets are involved in the pathogenesis of pre-eclampsia, and several small studies in the 1980s suggested that aspirin could prevent pre-eclampsia in those at risk [29]. Although some large, well-designed studies failed to confirm this early promise[30,31], a recent meta-analysis [32] of studies involving more than 30,000 women found that use of low dose aspirin was associated with a 10% reduction in both the diagnosis of pre-eclampsia (95% confidence intervals, 3–16%) and the numbers of infants born before 34 weeks (2–17%).

Antioxidants – Oxidative stress is believed to play a major role in pre-eclampsia. Recently, a large randomised placebo-controlled trial examined the efficacy of the antioxidants vitamins C and E in the prevention of pre-eclampsia. This study concluded that these vitamins were *not* associated with a reduction in the incidence of pre-eclampsia [33].

Key points

- ACE inhibitors and angiotensin II receptor antagonists are contraindicated in pregnancy
- β-Blockers are safe antihypertensive agents for use in the third trimester but may cause growth restriction if used in high doses from early in pregnancy
- Methyldopa is a safe antihypertensive for use throughout pregnancy
- Low dose aspirin can reduce the risk of pre-eclampsia, but its effect is modest.

Diuretics

Thiazide diuretics

These include *hydrochlorothiazide* and *bendroflumethazide*. They inhibit absorption of sodium and chloride in the distal renal tubule and lead to loss of potassium. They appear not to be teratogenic [15]. They cause a reduction in intravascular volume and although there is a theoretical risk of reduced uteroplacental perfusion leading to IUGR, this has never been demonstrated. When used long-term in pregnancy (usually for women with heart failure and/or pulmonary oedema), the mother's electrolytes should be checked regularly. Regular ultrasound scans are indicated to monitor for IUGR and oligohydramnios. If the mother has been given thiazides towards the end of pregnancy, the neonate is also at risk of electrolyte imbalance (hyponatraemia, hypocalcaemia) or hypoglycaemia (because of the diabetogenic effect on the mother).

Furosemide is a potent loop diuretic whose action wears off in 2–4 hours. Its only indications in pregnancy are cardiovascular disorders such as pulmonary oedema or heart failure; it should *not* be used for pre-eclampsia as it significantly reduces intravascular volume (thus exacerbating the intravascular depletion inherent in this condition). If used long-term, the decrease in plasma volume may lead to growth restriction in the fetus, although it does not seem to significantly decrease amniotic fluid volume [34]. Furosemide does not appear to be teratogenic.

Spironolactone is an aldosterone antagonist which leads to potassium retention. It does not appear to be teratogenic [15]; however, experience is limited, so it is relatively contraindicated in pregnancy. Spironolactone is known to have anti-androgenic effects and theoretically could cause feminisation of a male fetus, although this has not been reported.

Amiloride directly influences tubular transport and is a potassium-saving diuretic. It does not appear to be teratogenic [15]. However, as with spironolactone, data are lacking and the drug is relatively contraindicated in pregnancy.

Anti-arrhythmics

Minor arrhythmias and palpitations appear to be more common in pregnancy but generally do not need to be treated. However, if the effectiveness of the heart as a pump becomes impaired, treatment is important. Anti-arrhythmics are arranged in classes (1A, 1B, 1C, 2, 3 and 4) according to the effect they have on electrical conduction in the heart and the arrhythmia for which they are used [35].

Class 1A – This includes *disopyramide, quinidine and procainamide.* The last two are used relatively commonly in pregnancy and do not appear to be teratogenic [15]. In high doses, quinidine has an oxytoxic effect and may cause abortion [36], but in therapeutic doses it appears safe.

Class 1B – This includes *lidocaine, phenytoin* and others. Lidocaine has no teratogenic effects, but maternal lidocaine toxicity (e.g., hyperthermia) may also lead to fetal toxicity [37]. The teratogenic effects of phenytoin were first recognised back in 1964 [38] and are described in Chapter 9.

Class 1C – *Flecainide* has been used to treat fetal arrhythmias; it does not appear to be teratogenic or fetotoxic in humans.

Class 2 β-blockers – These have been considered earlier.

Class 3 – This includes *amiodarone, bretylium* and the β-*blocker sotalol.* Amiodarone has been used for both maternal and fetal arrhythmias. Although it contains high levels of iodine and can lead to congenital goitre or hypothyroidism [39], this seems to be transient [15]. Nevertheless, as data are limited, amiodarone should not be a first-line drug in pregnancy, either for maternal arrhythmia or for uncomplicated cases of fetal supraventricular tachycardia (SVT).

Sotalol has been used for both maternal and fetal arrhythmias. As with other β-blockers, it has the potential to cause IUGR, so serial ultrasound is indicated. Sotalol is effective in fetal atrial fibrillation (AF), but in fetal SVT the mortality rate is high and the conversion rate low, so the risks seem to outweigh the benefits. For maternal treatment, the risks and benefits must be weighed on an individual basis [40,41].

Class 4 – This includes the calcium antagonists *diltiazem* and *verapamil.* This class of drugs has been discussed earlier.

Electrical cardioversion

Direct current cardioversion appears to be safe and effective in pregnancy. Its use has been reported in pregnancy for the treatment of AF, atrial flutter and atrial tachycardia resistant to drug therapy [35,40].

Digoxin

Digoxin has been used successfully for the control of heart failure, atrial flutter and fibrillation, and no adverse effects on the fetus have been reported following therapeutic doses in pregnancy. Digoxin freely crosses the placenta [42] and has been shown to be effective in treating fetal SVT in utero [43–45]. Digoxin levels must be monitored during pregnancy as maternal toxicity may be fatal to the fetus; furthermore, renal clearance is increased as pregnancy advances, so the dose may need to be increased.

Nitrates

This group includes *glyceryl trinitrate, isosorbide mononitrate* and *isosorbide dinitrate*. Generally used as coronary dilators in ischaemic heart disease, they have also been used as tocolytics. Pregnancy data are limited, although their use is expected to increase as the average age of pregnancy, and hence the incidence of ischaemic heart disease, rises. However, they appear safe; occasional transient hypotension in the mother does not appear severe enough to significantly affect placental perfusion [15].

Anticoagulation

Many women with cardiac disease in pregnancy will require either thromboprophylaxis or full anticoagulation. Anticoagulation in pregnancy is described in detail in Chapter 4.

Key points

- In pregnancy, the diuretics of choice are the thiazides and furosemide
- The commonest arrhythmia in pregnancy is SVT
- Adenosine can be used to terminate SVT in pregnancy
- Cardioversion is safe in pregnancy
- Digoxin is safe and effective for AF, but toxic maternal levels can be fatal to the fetus

References

1 Schardein JL. *Chemically-Induced Birth Defects, 4th edition*. New York: Marcel Dekker; 2000.

2 Redman CWG, Beilin LJ, Bonnar J. Treatment of hypertension in pregnancy with methyldopa: blood pressure control and side effects. *Br J Obstet Gynaecol* 1977;**84**:419–26.

3 Jones HMR, Cummings AJ, Setchell KDR, Lawson AM. A study of the deposition of α-methyldopa in newborn infants following its administration to the mothers for the treatment of hypertension during pregnancy. *Br J Clin Pharmacol* 1979;**7**:433–40.

4 Whitelaw A. Maternal methyldopa treatment and neonatal blood pressure. *Br Med J* 1981;**283**:471.

5 Ounsted M, Cockburn J, Moar VA, Redman CWG. Maternal hypertension with superimposed preeclampsia: effects on child development at 7½ years. *Br J Obstet Gynaecol* 1983;**90**:644–9.

6 Marlettini MG, Crippa S, Morselli-Labate AN, et al. Randomized comparison of calcium antagonists and β-blockers in the treatment of pregnancy-induced hypertension. *Curr Ther Res* 1990;**48**(4):684–92.

7 Orlandi C, Marlettini MG, Cassani A, et al. Treatment of hypertension during pregnancy with the calcium antagonist verapamil. *Curr Ther Res* 1986;**39**(6):884–93.
8 Chidress CH, Katz VL. Nifedipine and its indications in obstetrics and gynecology. *Obstet Gynecol* 1994;**83**:616–24.
9 Carbonne B, Jannet D, Touboul C, Khelifati Y, Milliez J. Nicardipine treatment of hypertension during pregnancy. *Obstet Gynecol* 1993;**81**:908–14.
10 Allen J, Maigaard S, Forman A, et al. Acute effects of nitrendipine in pregnancyinduced hypertension. *Br J Obstet Gynaecol* 1987;**94**: 222–6.
11 Wide-Swensson DH, Ingemarsson I, Lunell N, et al. Calcium channel blockade (isradipine) in treatment of hypertension in pregnancy: a randomised placebocontrolled study. *Am J Obstet Gynecol* 1995;**173**: 872–8.
12 Magee LA, Schick B, Donnenfield AE, et al. The safety of calcium channel blockers in human pregnancy: a prospective multicenter cohort study. *Am J Obstet Gynecol* 1996;**174**:823–8.
13 Waisman GD, Mayorga LM, Camera MI, Vignolo CA, Martinotti A. Magnesium plus nifedipine: potentiation of hypotensive effect in preeclampsia? *Am J Obstet Gynecol* 1988;**159**:308–9.
14 The Magpie Trial Collaborative Group. Do women with pre-eclampsia, and their babies, benefit from magnesium sulphate? The Magpie Trial: a randomised placebo-controlled trial. *Lancet* 2002;**359**:1877–90.
15 Briggs GG, Freeman RK, Yaffe SJ. *Drugs in Pregnancy and Lactation, 5th edition*. Baltimore: Williams and Wilkins; 1998.
16 Easterling TR, Brateng D, Schmucker B, Brown Z, Millard SP. The prevention of pre-eclampsia; a randomized trial of atenolol in hyperdynamic patients before onset of hypertension. *Obstet Gynecol* 1999;**93**: 725–33.
17 Butters L, Kennedy S, Rubin PC. Atenolol in essential hypertension during pregnancy. *Br Med J* 1990;**301**:587–9.
18 Lydakis C, Lip GY, Beavers M, Beavers DG. Atenolol and fetal growth in pregnancies complicated by hypertension. *Am J Hypertens* 1999;**12**:541–7.
19 Magee LA, Duley L. Oral beta-blockers for mild to moderate hypertension during pregnancy. The Cochrane Database of Systematic Reviews 2003; Issue 3: Art No CD002863.
20 von Dadelszen P, Ornstein MP, Bull SB, Logan AG, Koren G, Magee LA. Fall in mean arterial pressure and fetal growth restriction in pregnancy hypertension: a meta-analysis. *Lancet* 2000;**355**:87–92.
21 Reynolds B, Butters L, Evans J, Adama T, Rubin PC. First year of life after the use of atenolol in pregnancy-associated hypertension. *Arch Dis Child* 1984;**59**:1061–3.
22 Rubin PC, Butters L, Kelman AW, Fitzsimons C, Reid JL. Labetalol disposition and concentration – effect relationships during pregnancy. *Br J Clin Pharmacol* 1983;**15**:465–70.

23 Cooper WO, Hernandez-Diaz S, Arbogast PG, et al. Major congenital malformations after first-trimester exposure to ACE inhibitors. *N Engl J Med* 2006;**354**:2443–51.

24 Brent RL, Beckman DA. Angiotensin-converting enzyme inhibitors: an embryopathic class of drugs with unique properties: information for clinical teratology counsellors. *Teratology* 1991;**43**:543–6.

25 Saji H, Yamanaka M, Hagiwara A, Ijira R. Losartan and fetal toxic effects. *Lancet* 2001;**357**:363.

26 Lubbe WF, Hodge JV. Combined alpha and beta receptor antagonism with prasozin and oxprenolol in control of severe hypertension in pregnancy. *N Z Med J* 1981;**94**:169–72.

27 Spinnato JA, Sibai BM, Anderson GD. Fetal distress after hydralazine therapy for severe pregnancy-induced hypertension. *South Med J* 1986;**79**:559–62.

28 Eclampsia Trial Collaborative Group. Which anticonvulsant for women with eclampsia? Evidence from the Collaborative Eclampsia trial. *Lancet* 1995;**345**:1455–63.

29 Rubin PC. Aspirin and preeclampsia. *Curr Obstet Gynaecol* 1994;**4**: 166–9.

30 Sibai BM, Caritis S, Thom E. Prevention of preeclampsia with low dose aspirin in healthy, nulliparous pregnant women. *N Engl J Med* 1993;**329**:1213–9.

31 CLASP Collaborative group. CLASP: a randomised trial of low dose aspirin for the prevention and treatment of preeclampsia among 9364 pregnant women. *Lancet* 1994;**343**:619–29.

32 Askie LM, Duley L, Henderson-Smart DJ, on behalf of the PARIS Collaborative Group. Antiplatelet agents for the prevention of pre-eclampsia: a meta-analysis of individual patient data. *Lancet* 2007;**369**:1791–8.

33 Poston L, Briley AL, Seed PT, Kelly FJ, Shennan AH. Vitamin C and vitamin E in pregnant women at risk for pre-eclampsia (VIP trial): randomised placebo-controlled trial. *Lancet* 2006;**367**:1145–54.

34 Votta RA, Parada OH, Windgrad RH, Alvarez OH, Tomassinni TL, Patoria A. Furosemide action on the creatinine concentration of amniotic fluid. *Am J Obstet Gynecol* 1975;**123**:621–4.

35 Jogler JA, Page RL. Treatment of cardiac arrhythmias during pregnancy. *Drug Saf* 1999;**20**:85–94.

36 Rotmensch HH, Rotmensch S, Elkayam U. Management of cardiac arrhythmias during pregnancy: current concepts. *Drugs* 1987;**33**:623–33.

37 Macaulay JH, Bond K, Steer PJ. Epidural analgesia in labor and fetal hyperthermia. *Obstet Gynecol* 1992;**80**:665–9.

38 Janz D, Fuchs V. Are anti-epileptic drugs powerful when given during pregnancy? *Ger Med Monogr* 1964;**9**:20–3.

39 Grosso S, Berardi R, Cioni M, Morgese G. Transient neonatal hypothyroidism after gestational exposure to amiodarone: a follow-up of two cases. *J Endocrinol Invest* 1998;**21**:699–702.

40 Oudijk MA, Michon MM, Kleinman CS, et al. Sotalol in the treatment of fetal dysrrhythmias. *Circulation* 2000;**101**:2721–6.
41 Brown CEL, Wendel GD. Cardiac arrhythmias during pregnancy. *Clin Obstet Gynecol* 1989;**32**:89–102.
42 Chan V, Tse TF, Wong V. Transfer of digoxin across the placenta and into breast milk. *Br J Obstet Gynaecol* 1978;**85**:605–9.
43 Harrigan JT, Kangos JT, Sikka A, et al. Successful treatment of fetal congestive heart failure secondary to tachycardia. *N Engl J Med* 1981;**304**:1527–9.
44 Hsieh Y, Lee C, Chang C, Tsai H, Yeh L, Tsai C. Successful prenatal digoxin therapy for Ebstein's anomaly with hydrops fetalis. A case report. *J Reprod Med* 1998;**43**:710–2.
45 Tikanoja T, Kirkinen P, Nikolajev K, Eresmaa L, Haring P. Familial atrial fibrillation with fetal onset. *Heart* 1998;**79**:195–7.

CHAPTER 6
Treatment of endocrine diseases

Anastasios Gazis

This chapter reviews the treatment of commoner thyroid, adrenal and pituitary disorders which may complicate pregnancy.

The thyroid gland

A healthy woman normally has 10–20 g of thyroid tissue and requires a daily intake of approximately 50 mcg of iodine to prevent goitre (enlargement of the thyroid). A minimum of 150 mcg daily is generally recommended to support adequate thyroid hormone production.

Within the thyroid gland, follicular cells trap iodide and transport it to a colloid core. Here, thyroid peroxidase catalyses the oxidation and attachment of iodide to tyrosyl residues of thyroglobulin from which thyroid hormones are generated. Approximately 100 mcg of thyroxine (T_4 – with four iodide residues) and 30 mcg of tri-iodothyronine (T_3 – with three iodide residues) are released from the thyroid gland every day under the influence of thyroid-stimulating hormone (TSH). TSH regulates both the trapping of iodide and the release of thyroid hormones. A tightly governed feedback loop responds to peripheral thyroid hormone concentrations and controls TSH release from the anterior pituitary gland.

Less than 0.5% of circulating thyroid hormone is 'free' in the peripheral circulation and available for immediate use. Approximately 80% is bound to thyroid-binding globulin (TBG), 10% to

---

Prescribing in Pregnancy, 4th edition. Edited by Peter Rubin and Margaret Ramsay,
 ISBN: 978-1-4051-4712-5.

transthyretin and 10% to albumin. Bound thyroid hormones act as a buffer to ensure a ready supply of free thyroid hormones to all cell types. T_4, the most abundant circulating thyroid hormone, is de-iodinated to T_3, which acts upon nuclear receptors to govern transcriptional changes within cells.

Thyroid physiology in pregnancy

Placental delivery of maternal thyroid hormones is necessary for normal fetal development, particularly for intellectual development. Though the fetal thyroid begins to function at 10–12 weeks of gestation, it synthesises thyroid hormones only from 18 to 20 weeks of gestation. Output increases towards term [1] but most circulating fetal thyroid hormones are maternally derived even in the third trimester.

During the first trimester, there are two significant changes to maternal thyroid physiology. Firstly, oestrogen stimulates thyroxine-binding globulin (TBG) production and inhibits its excretion. The resultant near doubling of TBG is associated with a significant increase in concentrations of total circulating T_4 and T_3 but little change in free hormone levels [2]. Secondly, human chorionic gonadotrophin (hCG) is a weak agonist of the TSH receptor and so stimulates production and release of thyroid hormones. hCG concentrations peak towards the end of the first trimester, causing transient mild hyperthyroidism in 10–20% of women. As this change is physiological, it does not generally require treatment.

Hypothyroidism in pregnancy

Maternal hypothyroidism is associated with obstetric complications such as preterm delivery and fetal loss. Adequate maternal thyroid hormone availability and placental thyroid hormone transfer are essential for normal fetal development.

The earliest identification of the association between maternal thyroid status and fetal intellectual development came from areas where endemic iodine deficiency with maternal and fetal hypothyroidism was associated with profound neurological deficit in infants. These profound deficits are absent in congenitally hypothyroid infants born to euthyroid mothers. However, a low maternal free thyroid hormone concentration at the end of the first trimester is associated with poor psychomotor development in the infant [3]. Inadequate exposure to thyroxine in the second and third trimesters of gestation (and the first few months after birth) is also associated with significant intellectual and sometimes neurological disability. A study looking at the intellectual development of 7-year-old children born of mothers with elevated TSH (mean 13.2 μL) but normal T_4 during pregnancy showed that 1 in 5 of this group had an IQ less than 85 compared with 1 in 20 of a control group with normal TSH [4].

In women treated with thyroxine for hypothyroidism, the physiological changes of pregnancy require an increase in thyroid hormone supplementation [5] of approximately one-third. In one study, the earliest gestation at which an increase in thyroid hormone dose was required was 5 weeks, with a median of 8 weeks [6]. Dose increases plateau at approximately 16 weeks of gestation. Current recommendations are to maintain maternal TSH between 0.5 and 2.0 μL. The gestation at which thyroxine requirements increase and the magnitude of the increase required are often underestimated. Some authors therefore recommend an increase in maternal thyroxine of 25–50 mcg daily as soon as pregnancy is confirmed [7].

Inadequate thyroxine therapy of maternal hypothyroidism is generally regarded as the major cause of syndromes of fetal hypothyroidism. However, studies in the United States [8] and other nations suggest that deficient maternal iodine intake may contribute to an inability of apparently healthy euthyroid mothers to up-regulate thyroxine production for pregnancy. In countries such as Japan where the diet is iodine replete, less than 0.5% of pregnant women have elevated TSH, whereas in the United States, prevalence is approximately 2.5%. Maternal iodine deficiency is associated with a decrease in the ratio of T_4 to T_3 released by the maternal thyroid gland. Though this maintains a normal maternal TSH, the fetal brain is largely dependent upon de-iodination of maternal T_4 for its supply of T_3. Maternal iodine deficiency may mask relative fetal hypothyroidism.

Prevention of fetal hypothyroidism requires an adequate intake of iodine and treatment of remaining cases of hypothyroidism in women of childbearing potential, both preconceptually and through pregnancy.

Hyperthyroidism in pregnancy

Hyperthyroidism affects approximately 0.2% of pregnancies. Significant maternal hyperthyroidism requires treatment because it is associated with increased rates of fetal loss, growth restriction, fetal hydrops and pre-eclampsia. The commonest cause is Graves' disease, though any cause of hyperthyroidism may present in pregnancy. Diagnostic and therapeutic strategies are restricted by an absolute need to avoid radio-isotopes, to avoid surgery if possible and to minimise the risk of other iatrogenic harm.

hCG and the thyroid

The physiological increase in hCG in the first trimester of pregnancy may be associated with transient maternal thyrotoxicosis and does not usually require treatment. Hyperemesis gravidarum may be associated with very high levels of hCG. Associated thyrotoxicosis may require treatment, though a low dose of an antithyroid drug is usually sufficient. This should then be withdrawn rapidly as hyperemesis resolves. Gestational trophoblastic disease is also associated with high serum hCG, nausea, vomiting and thyrotoxicosis.

Graves' disease

Graves' disease is caused by stimulation of maternal thyroidal TSH receptors by maternally derived antibodies. However, as pregnancy progresses, Graves' thyrotoxicosis usually improves and the dose of antithyroid drug can be reduced. Approximately one-third of women are able to stop antithyroid drugs in the third trimester of pregnancy [9]. It is uncertain why the titre of maternally derived stimulating antibodies either declines or is offset by an increase in the titre of maternal TSH-receptor-blocking antibodies [10].

Fetal thyrotoxicosis affects approximately 1% of mothers with Graves' disease. Stimulating and blocking antibodies both cross the placenta and can cause fetal thyrotoxicosis or hypothyroidism, once fetal TSH receptors become active at approximately 20 weeks of gestation. Maternal thyroid antibody titres may persist despite antithyroid drug treatment or maternal antenatal thyroid ablation. Maternal euthyroidism does not guarantee fetal euthyroidism, and vigilance for fetal or neonatal hyperthyroidism is needed. If the maternal TSH-receptor antibody titre is negative, the fetus does not seem to be at risk.

Postpartum thyroiditis

Up to 10% of women develop postpartum thyroiditis. Characteristically, this begins soon after delivery and may persist for 12–18 months. A period of hyperthyroidism is followed by either euthyroidism or a period of hypothyroidism prior to re-establishment of a euthyroid state. Some women require β-blockade to counter adrenergic symptoms during the thyrotoxic phase and some require thyroxine treatment to counter hypothyroid symptoms. In general, thyroxine treatment is tapered over 6 months to determine whether hypothyroidism is permanent. This can occur if, for example, the hypothyroidism is not due to postnatal thyroiditis, but an alternative diagnosis such as Hashimoto's thyroiditis.

Antithyroid drug choice in pregnancy

If an antithyroid drug is used, it should be at the lowest dose and for the shortest duration possible. Maternal TSH should be maintained towards the bottom of the reference range and T_4 towards the top as mild thyrotoxicosis is less harmful to fetal development than hypothyroidism. As antithyroid drugs cross the placenta, frequent assessment of maternal thyroid status – perhaps 4–6 weekly – is needed to minimise antithyroid drug doses and reduce the risk of iatrogenic fetal hypothyroidism. A 'block and replace' regimen cannot be used because of the transplacental transfer of antithyroid drugs.

There are no large prospective randomised trials in pregnancy that compare the thionamide drugs, propylthiouracil and carbimazole (methimazole). Available data [11] demonstrate that though both drugs cross the placenta, fetal thyroid function at birth is not different whether propylthiouracil or carbimazole has been used [12]. Two congenital defects have given rise to concern in infants exposed to thionamide drugs. The first, aplasia cutis, is a minor congenital defect characterised by single or multiple small skin lesions on the fetal scalp. It occurs spontaneously in approximately 1 in 2000 births and there are case reports in infants exposed to methimazole [13], but none in infants exposed to propylthiouracil. Secondly, choanal or oesophageal atresia was found in 2 of 241 infants exposed to methimazole during pregnancy in one study [14]. At least one case of choanal atresia has been reported in an infant whose mother was exposed to propylthiouracil [11]. Despite the lack of robust data, propylthiouracil is becoming the drug of choice in pregnancy. Where propylthiouracil is not available or cannot be used for any reason, carbimazole (methimazole) is an acceptable alternative.

Thionamides are excreted in breast milk, methimazole to a greater degree than propylthiouracil. However, the quantities are too low to adversely affect the infant's thyroid function or intellectual development [15] and both can be used in breastfeeding mothers.

The adrenal glands

Hypoadrenalism

Primary (adrenal) hypoadrenalism is the commonest cause of hypoadrenalism in pregnancy and generally requires treatment before conception is possible. It is usually associated with mineralocorticoid deficiency that requires replacement with the potent synthetic mineralocorticoid, fludrocortisone.

Glucocorticoid and mineralocorticoid replacement does not usually require adjustment during pregnancy. Some women require modest upward adjustment of glucocorticoid replacement in the third trimester. Labour and delivery exert sufficient physiological stress to require supplementary glucocorticoid treatment. It is usual to give 100-mg intramuscular hydrocortisone at the onset of labour. If labour is prolonged, a continuous saline infusion with 25–50 mg of hydrocortisone every 6 hours may be required. Glucocorticoid doses should be doubled for 24–48 hours after delivery and then rapidly tapered (http://www.adshg.org.uk/comms/publications/surgicalguidelines-colour.pdf).

Congenital adrenal hyperplasia

Glucocorticoid and mineralocorticoid treatment in women who have congenital adrenal hyperplasia generally does not require adjustment through pregnancy. There is little evidence to support repeated assessment of the maternal androgen profile to adjust treatment as the fetus is protected from maternal androgens by placental aromatase.

At delivery, glucocorticoid treatment should be adjusted in the same way as for women requiring supplementation for primary hypoadrenalism. In some women with congenital adrenal hyperplasia, vaginal delivery can cause significant damage to the birth canal if it is not anatomically normal or if there has been previous surgery. Elective caesarean section may be preferable in these mothers.

The pituitary gland

Hypopituitarism

Hypopituitarism does not preclude pregnancy, but the lack of gonadotrophins prevents normal ovulation. Preparation for pregnancy should include the cessation of growth hormone treatment as its effect on a fetus is uncertain. Ovulation induction and/or assisted conception are necessary to establish pregnancy. The fetoplacental unit is then relatively self-sustaining, though replacement and adjustment of maternal thyroid and glucocorticoid hormones is necessary as it is for women with primary hypoadrenalism and hypothyroidism. Hypopituitarism is associated with undetectable or low TSH and precludes its use in assessing the adequacy of replacement.

Prolactinoma

Hyperprolactinaemia usually requires treatment to permit ovulation and conception. Prolactinoma is also associated with risks to mother from enlargement of the adenoma and/or pituitary and, to a lesser extent, the fetus from dopaminergic drugs.

Normal pregnancy is associated with an approximate doubling in pituitary size. In the mother, the hyperoestrogenic state of pregnancy specifically stimulates expansion of prolactin-secreting cells (lactotrophs). In a woman with prolactinoma, this may cause headache or more serious pressure symptoms such as secondary hormone deficiencies or visual loss if there is sufficient enlargement.

A *microprolactinoma* (<10 mm in diameter) is extremely unlikely to cause permanent or serious problems. The risk of symptoms such as headache in the mother is of the order of 1 or 2% and visual loss or secondary hormone deficiency is extremely unlikely. It is usual to review the mother during each trimester to assess clinically for symptoms of expansion. Where expansion of the prolactinoma causes serious pressure symptoms, a dopamine agonist is used, but this will be at the expense of breastfeeding as milk production is reliant upon the normal physiological rise in maternal prolactin.

A *macroprolactinoma* (>10 mm in diameter) carries a greater risk of problems during pregnancy. Approximately 40% of mothers develop pressure symptoms and 25% or more develop visual impairment. Where pregnancy is desired, the mother should be treated prior to pregnancy to shrink the adenoma as much as possible. The dopaminergic agent is usually stopped, once pregnancy is confirmed. The mother requires careful monitoring. Visual fields are usually assessed every trimester and pituitary MRI ordered if there are significant symptoms or signs. Dopaminergic therapy may need to be restarted. Pituitary surgery in pregnancy should be avoided, if possible.

The risk to the fetus from a dopaminergic drug used to treat hyperprolactinaemia is minimal if it is stopped once pregnancy is confirmed. The dopaminergic drugs bromocriptine or cabergoline are generally preferred in women who may become pregnant. Data from 1410 pregnancies suggest that the risks of spontaneous abortion and fetal malformation were not increased in women who took bromocriptine during the first month of pregnancy [16]. Similar data exist from a smaller study of women who took cabergoline for the first month of pregnancy [17]. Bromocriptine is generally used as first-line and cabergoline as second-line therapy. Pergolide is not used as it may be associated with cardiac valvular defects.

References

1 Thorpe-Beeston J, Nicolaides K, Felton C, Butler J, McGregor A. Maturation of the secretion of thyroid hormone and thyroid-stimulating hormone in the fetus. *N Engl J Med* 1991;**324**:532–6.

2 Burrow GN, Fisher DA, Larsen PR. Maternal and fetal thyroid function. *N Engl J Med* 1994;**331**:1072–8.

3 Pop VJ, Kuijpens JL, van Baar AL, et al. Low maternal free thyroxine concentrations during early pregnancy are associated with impaired psychomotor development in infancy. *Clin Endocrinol* 1999;**50**:149–55.

4 Haddow JE, Palomaki GE, Allan WC, et al. Maternal thyroid deficiency during pregnancy and subsequent neuropsychological development of the child. *N Engl J Med* 1999;**341**:549–55.

5 Mandel S, Larsen P, Seely E, Brent G. Increased need for thyroxine during pregnancy in women with primary hypothyroidism. *N Engl J Med* 1990;**323**:91–6.

6 Alexander EK, Marqusee E, Lawrence J, Jarolim P, Fischer GA, Larsen PR. Timing and magnitude of increases in levothyroxine requirements during pregnancy in women with hypothyroidism. *N Engl J Med* 2004;**351**: 241–9.

7 Toft A. Increased levothyroxine requirements in pregnancy – why, when, and how much? *N Engl J Med* 2004;**351**:292–4.

8 Hollowell JG, Staehling NW, Hannon WH, et al. Iodine nutrition in the United States. Trends and public health implications: iodine excretion data from National Health and Nutrition Examination Surveys I and III (1971–1974 and 1988–1994). *J Clin Endocrinol Metab* 1998;**83**:3401–8.

9 Weetman AP. Graves' Disease. *N Engl J Med* 2000;**343**:1236–48.

10 Kung AWC, Jones BM. A change from stimulatory to blocking antibody activity in Graves' disease during pregnancy. *J Clin Endocrinol Metab* 1998;**83**:514–8.

11 Cheron RG, Kaplan MM, Larsen PR, Selenkow HA, Crigler JF. Neonatal thyroid function after propylthiouracil therapy for maternal Graves' disease. *N Engl J Med* 1981;**304**:525–8.

12 Momotani N, Noh J, Oyanagi H, Ishikawa N, Ito K. Antithyroid drug therapy for Graves' disease during pregnancy. Optimal regimen for fetal thyroid status. *N Engl J Med* 1986;**315**:24–8.

13 Mandel SJ, Brent GA, Lasson PR. Review of antithyroid drug use during pregnancy and report of a case of aplasia cutis. *Thyroid* 1994;**4**:129–33.

14 Di Gianantonio E, Schaefer C, Mastroiacovo P, et al. Adverse effects of prenatal methimazole exposure. *Teratology* 2001;**64**:262–6.

15 Azizi F, Khoshniat M, Bahrainian M, Hedayati M. Thyroid function and intellectual development of infants nursed by mothers taking methimazole. *J Clin Endocrinol Metab* 2000;**85**:3233–8.

16 Turkalj I, Braun P, Krupp P. Surveillance of bromocriptine in pregnancy. *JAMA* 1982;**247**:1589–91.

17 Robert E, Musatti L, Piscitelli G, Ferrari CI. Pregnancy outcome after treatment with the ergot derivative, cabergoline. *Reprod Toxicol* 1996;**10**: 333–7.

CHAPTER 7
Drugs in rheumatic disease during pregnancy

Mary Gayed, Caroline Gordon

Introduction

Many rheumatological diseases will present in women during childbearing years. This often necessitates the use of antirheumatic therapy to allow the disease process to be brought under control, and so pregnancy can be achieved and maintained to term. Despite the natural inclination of patients to reduce or stop as many drugs as possible during pregnancy and lactation, disease activity must be controlled and drug therapy should be reduced to the minimum possible dose, to provide the least possible risk to mother and baby but without risking adverse events due to disease flare. Patients need pre-pregnancy counselling to ensure that they are taking appropriate drugs prior to and during early pregnancy. Such counselling should include advice about the risks of disease flare and other complications that may occur in pregnancy and the consequences of this for the mother and baby.

Analgesia

Simple analgesics are commonly used for musculoskeletal pain and are easily obtained over the counter. They are used in pregnancy by women regardless of whether or not they have a rheumatic disease and are fully described in Chapter 2 and are summarised in Table 7.1.

Prescribing in Pregnancy, 4th edition. Edited by Peter Rubin and Margaret Ramsay,
 ISBN: 978-1-4051-4712-5.

Table 7.1 Risks of drugs used in rheumatic diseases for pregnancy and lactation

	Main use in rheumatic diseases	Possible risks to fetus	Contraindicated in pregnancy	Contraindicated in lactation	Fertility impairment
		Analgesic, anti-inflammatory and antithrombotic drugs			
Paracetamol	Analgesia	Unlikely	No	No	Not known
Codeine	Analgesia	Respiratory depression, withdrawal syndrome	No – caution needed	No – caution needed	Not known
Aspirin	Antithrombotic	Very low risk with small doses, high doses are associated with neonatal haemorrhage and pulmonary hypertension	No – low-dose recommended	No – low-dose recommended	Not known
Heparin and low-molecular-weight heparin	Antithrombotic	No evidence	No	No	Not known
NSAIDS (in general)	Analgesia	Late pregnancy – constriction of ductus arteriosis	Caution needed in first and third trimester	See below	Inhibition of cilia in fallopian tube
Ibuprofen	Example of mild NSAID	Late pregnancy – constriction of ductus arteriosis	Caution needed in first and third trimester	No – low doses	Cases of inhibition of follicle rupture

(Continued)

Table 7.1 *(Continued)*

	Main use in rheumatic diseases	Possible risks to fetus	Contraindicated in pregnancy	Contraindicated in lactation	Fertility impairment
Indomethacin	Example of potent NSAID, used in spondylitis	Miscarriages, congenital malformations, prolonged gestation, pulmonary hypertension	Yes	Yes	Cases of inhibition of follicle rupture
		Antirheumatic drugs			
Hydroxychloroquine	RA, SLE	Not at recommended doses	No – low dose	No – low dose	Not studied
Sulphasalazine	RA, spondy-loarthropathies	Aplastic anaemia in maternal dose > 2 g; folate supplements recommended	No	No – avoid high dose	In men: oligospermia, reduce sperm mobility and abnormal forms
Gold	RA	None confirmed	No – low dose	No – low dose	Not studied
Leflunomide	RA, SLE	Congenital abnormalities; washout needed before planned pregnancy	Yes	Yes	Not studied
Penicillamine	RA	Connective tissue disease	Yes	Yes	Not studied
		Immunosuppressive drugs			
Prednisolone	SLE, RA, vasculitis	Rare (cataract, cleft palate, infection, infection)	No – caution needed with high doses	No – caution needed with high doses	Not studied

Methotrexate	RA, SLE, psoriasis	Cytopenia, facial and skeletal abnormalities	Yes	Yes	Yes, at high dose in women and oligospermia in men
Cyclosporin	RA, SLE, vasculitis	Transient immune alterations, growth retardations	No – low dose	No – caution needed	No
Azathioprine	RA, SLE, vasculitis	Sporadic congenital abnormalities, transient immune alterations	No – caution needed with high dose	Conflicting evidence	No
Mycophenolate	SLE, vasculitis	Multiple fetal abnormalities	Yes	Yes	Not studied
Cyclophosphamide	SLE, vasculitis	Chromosomal abnormalities, cytopenia	Yes	Yes	Gonadotoxic in both sexes
		Biological agents			
Etanercept	RA	Insufficient data available	Yes	Yes	Not studied
Infliximab	RA	Insufficient data available	Yes	Yes	Not studied
Rituximab	RA, SLE	No data available	Yes	Yes	Not studied

Aspirin

Aspirin is rarely used now in the treatment of inflammatory arthritis, but it is still a commonly used over-the-counter medication. When used at therapeutic analgesic dose, aspirin probably has a risk of miscarriages and infertility as do other NSAIDS (see Chapter 2). This is in contrast to low-dose aspirin taken by patients with recurrent fetal loss due to antiphospholipid syndrome in whom miscarriage risk may be reduced by aspirin (either alone or in combination with heparin) [1]. Low-dose aspirin may also be used as an anti-platelet agent and to reduce the risk of pre-eclampsia during pregnancy in women with systemic lupus erythematosus (SLE) and other high-risk pregnancies [1]. Exposure to aspirin in pregnancy has not been associated with any significant increase in congenital abnormalities or minor physical anomalies in infants [2].

Corticosteroids

Corticosteroids are used mostly to control maternal systemic rheumatic diseases such as SLE and vasculitis, but are sometimes used to help control inflammatory arthritis and in pregnancy, spondylitis. Less than 10% of oral prednisolone (and prednisone) administered to the mother reaches the fetus as the enzyme 11-β-hydroxysteroid dehydrogenase in the placenta converts cortisol and corticosterone to the relatively inactive 11-keto forms. Therefore it appears to be safe to use these drugs (and even intravenous methylprednisolone) in women who require corticosteroids to control rheumatic (and other inflammatory) diseases during pregnancy [3]. They are the treatment of choice for lupus and vasculitis flares, and prednisolone or intra-articular methylprednisolone may be useful for arthritic flares and spondyloarthropathies that are troublesome in pregnancy. These corticosteroids are safer than high-dose NSAIDs and can be used in all trimesters of pregnancy. In the humans, they may lead to a very small increase of oral clefts or cleft palate from exposure to hydrocortisone and prednisone during the first trimester of pregnancy. However, a reporting bias might exist since several large studies have found no statistically increased rate of oral clefts. Current data suggest that embryonic exposure to corticosteroids might increase the rate of oral cleft from 1 per 1000 births in the general population to about 3 per 1000 births, but no other congenital abnormalities have been reported in those exposed to steroids inactivated by 11-β-hydroxysteroid dehydrogenase [4].

Disease-modifying antirheumatic drugs

Antimalarial drugs

Chloroquine and hydroxychloroquine are antimalarial agents that are used as second-line agents in the management of SLE and RA (rheumatoid arthritis). It is now recommended to maintain hydroxychloroquine treatment during pregnancy and lactation, as it will reduce the risk of maternal disease flare and associated complications and it has not been shown to cause any fetal damage [4,5]. Chloroquine is rarely used now because of its increased risk of retinal toxicity in the non-pregnant woman, and patients taking it should be changed to hydroxychloroquine before they become pregnant. There are no data on the use of mepacrine in pregnancy and lactation, so it cannot be recommended.

Treatment at the correct therapeutic dose of 200–400 mg daily of hydroxychloroquine has not been found to increase the incidence of congenital abnormalities [6–8]. Despite theoretical risks of toxicity from hydroxychloroquine exposure in utero and during lactation, it has not been found to cause reduced visual acuity, or abnormalities in visual fields, colour field defects, electroretinogram and electro-oculogram abnormalities, secondary to corneal deposition or pigmentary retinopathy [9,10]. Hydroxychloroquine has been associated with a higher rate of preterm delivery than the general population, but this is most likely to be attributed to underlying disease in the mother for which the drug was prescribed [9]. Recent evidence suggests that it also has antithrombotic properties that may be particularly beneficial in patients with antiphospholipid antibodies [11].

Sulphasalazine

Sulphasalazine has been demonstrated to be a safe drug in pregnancy and lactation, when studied in pregnant women with RA or inflammatory bowel disease [12,13]. However, some experts have advised that sulphasalazine should be avoided in the last trimester, because of the theoretical risk of pathological jaundice due to the displacement of bilirubin from albumin, but there have been no reports of kernicterus in the newborn. When levels of sulphasalazine have been measured in cord blood, the levels were found to be negligible, and thus the bilirubin displacing capacity seems to be very low [14]. Aplastic anaemia has been reported in an aborted fetus with first-trimester exposure to sulphasalazine. There has also been a case of neutropenia in an infant whose mother took 3 g daily during pregnancy [15,16], but these are rare events. Sulphasalazine has been found to be safe to be used in lactating women. There has been one report of neonatal diarrhoea, which was attributed to an increased dose during the mothers' therapy [17]. Folate supplements are recommended before and during pregnancy, as sulphasalazine impairs folate absorption [18].

Gold

There are limited reports of gold use in pregnancy. Rheumatologists usually recommend that women of childbearing age on gold preparations should use adequate contraception. It has been suggested that if given monthly as maintenance therapy, each injection of gold should be timed with the start of menses. Thus it is easy to withdraw gold therapy if menses are delayed and the patient suspects pregnancy [19]. Gold compounds cross the placenta and have been found in the liver and kidneys of aborted fetuses, but there is no hard evidence regarding the teratogenic effects of gold therapy (intramuscular or oral) in pregnancy [20–22]. Because of the lack of evidence, it has been recommended that the dose and frequency of gold injections are reduced to the minimum possible, and usually monthly dose has been sufficient to maintain disease control in pregnancy, given that arthritis usually improves in pregnancy. The alternative approach is to discontinue gold injections when pregnancy is diagnosed. However, many rheumatologists have preferred to leave patients on intermittent gold injections to minimise the risk of flares of arthritis during or after pregnancy. Even though the risks of continuing therapy are low, women should be appropriately counselled and monitored closely during pregnancy [19].

Gold is excreted in breast milk and is absorbed by the infant. There have been a few reports of rash, nephritis, hepatitis and haematological problems in the newborn, but no cause–effect relationship has been established [19,23]. Thus it is recommended to breastfeed with caution or not at all, due to the potential risk of gold toxicity in the infant [23], but in practice, as gold is now rarely used for the management of rheumatic diseases, this is an infrequent problem.

Leflunomide

Leflunomide is a new and effective recently approved disease-modifying antirheumatic drug for the treatment of RA. Leflunomide is contraindicated in pregnancy and lactation, and a reliable and safe contraceptive therapy is recommended for men and women receiving leflunomide. Female patients should have a negative pregnancy test before commencing therapy as it is known to be teratogenic [24,25]. The additional concern regarding leflunomide is its extremely long half-life. The active metabolite has been detected for up to 2 years following cessation of the drug administration unless a regimen of cholestyramine is initiated [19, 25] to promote rapid leflunomide. If high levels persist, further cholestyramine may be given [19,25]. Currently, there is little human data about the fetal and neonatal effects of leflunomide exposure during pregnancy.

Penicillamine

Penicillamine is a chelating agent used in the treatment of RA, systemic sclerosis and Wilson's disease. The use of penicillamine is contraindicated in pregnancy, as fetal exposure has been found to cause connective tissue diseases, hernias and growth retardation [26]. It is advised to stop penicillamine before conception or as soon as pregnancy has been confirmed, and it should be avoided in lactation. The only exception is Wilson's disease, where the benefits outweigh the risk as penicillamine is needed to provide fetal protection from excess maternal copper levels [27,28].

Methotrexate

Methotrexate is a folic acid antagonist, used in the treatment of RA, SLE, vasculitis and psoriasis; It is contraindicated in pregnancy as it is highly teratogenic [24]. The active metabolites remain in cells or tissues several months after discontinuation, so it should be stopped 3–6 months prior to planned conception, in both men and women. It should be noted that the embryo is the most susceptible to the metabolites at week 5 when the closure of the neural tube takes place [29]. It is essential to continue folic acid supplements, even after the withdrawal of methotrexate in women planning and undergoing pregnancy.

Experience with methotrexate during pregnancy is mainly derived from oncology patients taking methotrexate, or following unsuccessful use of methotrexate to terminate pregnancy [30,31].

In these cases the methotrexate doses were higher than the once-weekly doses of about 10 mg, recommended when treating RA. In the case of the oncology patients the fetus would have been exposed to more than one chemotherapy agent [31]. Results from these studies have demonstrated multiple anomalies in infants, including anencephaly, hydrocephalic and meningomyelocele.

There have been 63 cases of methotrexate use in the first trimester pregnancy for the treatment of rheumatological conditions at a weekly dose of 20 mg or less [4]. In the pregnancies where termination was not sought, 11 of the pregnancies resulted in miscarriage, 33 proceeded to delivery, of which 4 had congenital abnormalities [4].

Methotrexate is contraindicated in lactation, as it is secreted into breast milk in small amounts. The milk-to-plasma ratio is 0.08, but potential accumulation may occur, causing immune suppression, neutropenia and carcinogenesis [19,32].

Cyclosporin

Cyclosporin is used in the treatment of RA, SLE, vasculitis and in transplant recipients. Approximately 800 cases of pregnancy in patients on cyclosporin have been reported, the majority of which were in transplant recipients [4,33,34].

No specific pattern of congenital anomalies has been identified, and the incident rate is 3%, which does not exceed that of the general population [4]. There is an increased but not significant rate of prematurity and low birth weight, but it is not clear if this is due to the cyclosporin therapy or the underlying maternal disease requiring the therapy [4].

Cyclosporin is considered safe for use in pregnancy after appropriate counselling at the lowest possible dose. There have been 15 reported cases of breastfeeding without any side effects, but breastfeeding is not recommended, as it is secreted to breast milk and may cause immunosuppressive and other effects in the baby [4,35].

Azathioprine

This is a cytotoxic immunosuppressant used to treat SLE, inflammatory bowel disease, haematological malignancies and renal transplant patients. The fetus is thought to be protected from the potential teratogenic effects of the drug as the fetus lacks the enzyme inosinatopyrophophorylase that is required to convert azathioprine to active metabolite 6-MP [36].

Azathioprine can be used in pregnancy to control severe maternal disease. The maximum recommended dose is 2 mg/kg [4]. Side effects of maternal therapy on the fetus are rare but there have been some reports of intrauterine growth restriction, transient chromosomal anomalies, adrenal hypoplasia and reduced serum immunoglobulin levels [19,37,38]. Decreased haematopoiesis was reported in infants whose mothers were treated with doses exceeding 2 mg/kg daily [39]. However, studies of normal pregnancy and delivery of healthy neonates have been reported in many women with SLE, inflammatory bowel disease and renal transplantation treated with azathioprine during pregnancy [4,40–42].

Breastfeeding is not widely recommended as low doses of azathioprine (0.1% of the maternal dose) are found in breast milk. This might lead to long-term potential immunosuppression and carcinogenesis, but this has not been reported to date. Some units do continue low-dose azathioprine in the lactating mother due to the high risk of postpartum flare in rheumatic and other inflammatory diseases and the absence of adverse effects on the child [4].

Mycophenolate mofetil

Mycophenolate mofetil is an immunosuppressive drug used in the treatment of vasculitis, SLE and post-transplant patients. It is contraindicated in pregnancy and should only be given in women and men of childbearing age with reliable contraception. The recommendation is that mycophenolate mofetil should be stopped at least 6 months before pregnancy is achieved, due to its long half-life and enterohepatic recirculation.

There are no controlled studies on pregnancy during treatment with mycophenolate mofetil. Data that are available from drug company files and the National Transplantation Pregnancy Registry suggest that there is an increased risk of congenital abnormalities, but no specific phenotype has been identified [4]. Breastfeeding is contraindicated for women taking mycophenolate mofetil, as there are no existing data on excretion in breast milk and it is potentially cytotoxic in the newborn.

Cyclophosphamide

Cyclophosphamide is used in the treatment of SLE and vasculitis. Fertility is an important issue in its use in women and men hoping to have children, as there is a significant risk of infertility that increases with the age at first dose and the total accumulated dose whether given orally or as intravenous infusions (pulses) [43]. When taken orally daily, permanent ovarian failure develops in more than 70% of women [19], but the risk is less with intermittent intravenous infusions.

Cyclophosphamide is contraindicated during pregnancy, as it is teratogenic. The risk of structural deformities is highest in the first trimester; reports of anomalies of craniofacial anomalies and growth retardation have been made [44]. However, the rate of miscarriage or congenital anomalies was not found to be increased in women who had completed courses of cyclophosphamide therapy prior to pregnancy [45]. It is recommended that women should not become pregnant for at least 3 months after discontinuing cyclophosphamide. There have been occasional reports of intravenous cyclophosphamide treatment for life-threatening vasculitis and lupus nephritis in the mother in the third trimester of pregnancy [1,46]. This has been associated with a high risk of intrauterine growth restriction and stillbirth, probably due to the combined effects of the disease and the drug. Delivery of the fetus before the institution of cytotoxic therapy is usually preferable, since the disease is often easier to control after delivery, and this approach avoids the neonate being exposed to the drug. High-dose oral steroids or intravenous methylprednisolone infusions appear to be safer for the fetus, although there is very little data and there are no controlled trials.

Breastfeeding is contraindicated during cyclophosphamide therapy, as cyclophosphamide is found in substantial concentrations in breast milk, and suppression of haematopoiesis has been reported in a breastfed infant [4,47].

Biological agents

Etanercept

Etanercept is a tumour necrosis factor antagonist, used in the treatment of patients with moderate to severe RA, who do not adequately respond to one or more disease-modifying antirheumatic drugs. At present it is contraindicated in pregnancy, as there is little data on its effects during pregnancy. There has been a report of a woman with psoriatic arthritis on etanercept, 50 mg twice weekly, giving birth to a child with VATER (vertebrae anomalies, anal anomalies, tracheal problems, oesophageal problems, radial or renal defects) association [48]. However, there have been other reports suggesting no increased risk of congenital anomalies or other adverse effects in pregnant women taking etanercept. At present it is not known whether or not teratogenesis is dose related [4]. Breastfeeding is also contraindicated, as like many drugs and immunoglobulins it has been shown to be secreted in breast milk, and the potential side effects for the fetus are unknown [4].

Infliximab

Infliximab is also contraindicated in pregnancy and lactation, because of the lack of evidence available, and should be stopped as soon as pregnancy is confirmed. Studies have been carried out looking at both women with Crohn's disease and RA who became pregnant while taking infliximab. In one study it was found that pregnancy outcomes did not differ from that of a healthy control group. Complications that were observed included prematurity and tetralogy of Fallot [25]. In a more recent analysis of 96 women exposed to Infliximab during pregnancy, five infants were born with complications including tetralogy of Fallot, intestinal malformations and respiratory distress [48].

Rituximab

At present there are no data on the effects of fetal exposure to rituximab (anti-CD 20 monoclonal antibody) therapy given to the mother prior to or during pregnancy. The drug company recommends discontinuing the drug 12 months before planning pregnancy as B-cell depletion in the mother can last over 6 months. Similarly there are no data on the excretion of rituximab in breast milk and breastfeeding should cease before therapy is started.

Conclusion

Prior to pregnancy it is important to counsel the mother on the effects of her rheumatic disease on pregnancy and those of the pregnancy on the disease. She will need detailed advice about the use of antirheumatic and analgesic therapies during conception, pregnancy and lactation, and their potential benefits and complications. It is important to establish control of disease activity before she conceives, preferably on appropriate drugs that can be continued in pregnancy. It should not be forgotten that women may be taking other medications, such as ACE inhibitors for hypertension or proteinuria and proton pump inhibitors for dyspepsia, which will also need to be discussed and changed preferably before conception occurs. With coordinated management between the rheumatologist, obstetrician and any other physician involved in the care of patients with systemic manifestations of rheumatic disease, most women can now have successful pregnancies.

References

1 Gordon C. Pregnancy and autoimmune diseases. *Best Pract Res Clin Rheumatol* 2004;**18**(3):359–79.
2 Bonaminio PN, de Regnier R, Chang E, Day N, Manzi S, Ramsey-Goldman R. Minor physical anomalies are not increased in the offspring of mothers with systemic lupus erythematosus. *Ann Rheum Dis* 2006;**65**(2):246–8.
3 Clowse M, Petri M. Pregnancy and SLE. In: Tsokos G, Gordon C, Smolen J (eds.), *Systemic Lupus Erythematosus: A Companion to Rheumatology, 1st edition*. Philadelphia: Mosby Elsevier; 2007:449–59.
4 Ostensen M, Khamashta M, Lockshin M, et al. Anti-inflammatory and immunosuppressive drugs and reproduction. *Arthritis Res Ther* 2006;**8**(3):209.
5 Clowse ME, Magder L, Witter F, Petri M. Hydroxychloroquine in lupus pregnancy. *Arthritis Rheum* 2006;**54**(11):3640–7.
6 Costedoat-Chalumeau N, Amoura Z, Aymard G, et al. Evidence of transplacental passage of hydroxychloroquine in humans. *Arthritis Rheum* 2002;**46**(4):1123–4.
7 Buchanan NM, Toubi E, Khamashta MA, Lima F, Kerslake S, Hughes GR. Hydroxychloroquine and lupus pregnancy: review of a series of 36 cases. *Ann Rheum Dis* 1996;**55**(7):486–8.
8 Costedoat-Chalumeau N, Amoura Z, Duhaut P, et al. Safety of hydroxychloroquine in pregnant patients with connective tissue diseases: a study of one hundred thirty-three cases compared with a control group. *Arthritis Rheum* 2003;**48**(11):3207–11.
9 Motta M, Tincani A, Faden D, et al. Follow-up of infants exposed to hydroxychloroquine given to mothers during pregnancy and lactation. *J Perinatol* 2005;**25**(2):86–9.
10 Klinger G, Morad Y, Westall CA, et al. Ocular toxicity and antenatal exposure to chloroquine or hydroxychloroquine for rheumatic diseases. *Lancet* 2001;**358**(9284):813–4.
11 Pierangeli SS, Chen PP, Gonzalez EB. Antiphospholipid antibodies and the antiphospholipid syndrome: an update on treatment and pathogenic mechanisms. *Curr Opin Hematol* 2006;**13**(5):366–75.

12 Norgard B, Czeizel AE, Rockenbauer M, Olsen J, Sorensen HT. Population-based case control study of the safety of sulfasalazine use during pregnancy. *Aliment Pharmacol Ther* 2001;**15**(4):483–6.
13 Nielsen OH, Andreasson B, Bondesen S, Jarnum S. Pregnancy in ulcerative colitis. *Scand J Gastroenterol* 1983;**18**(6):735–42.
14 Jarnerot G, Andersen S, Esbjorner E, Sandstrom B, Brodersen R. Albumin reserve for binding of bilirubin in maternal and cord serum under treatment with sulphasalazine. *Scand J Gastroenterol* 1981;**16**(8): 1049–55.
15 Zwi LJ, Becroft DM. Intrauterine aplastic anemia and fetal hydrops: a case report. *Pediatr Pathol* 1986;**5**(2):199–205.
16 Levi S, Liberman M, Levi AJ, Bjarnason I. Reversible congenital neutropenia associated with maternal sulphasalazine therapy. *Eur J Pediatr* 1988;**148**(2):174–5.
17 Branski D, Kerem E, Gross-Kieselstein E, Hurvitz H, Litt R, Abrahamov A. Bloody diarrhea – a possible complication of sulfasalazine transferred through human breast milk. *J Pediatr Gastroenterol Nutr* 1986;**5**(2):316–7.
18 Hernandez-Diaz S, Werler MM, Walker AM, Mitchell AA. Folic acid antagonists during pregnancy and the risk of birth defects. *N Engl J Med* 2000;**343**(22):1608–14.
19 Janssen NM, Genta MS. The effects of immunosuppressive and anti-inflammatory medications on fertility, pregnancy, and lactation. *Arch Intern Med* 2000;**160**(5):610–9.
20 Richards AJ, Henderson W. Transfer of gold from mother to foetus. *Lancet* 1977;**1**:99.
21 Cohen DL, Orzel J, Taylor A. Infants of mothers receiving gold therapy. *Arthritis Rheum* 1981;**24**(1):104–5.
22 Ostensen M, Husby G. Antirheumatic drug treatment during pregnancy and lactation. *Scand J Rheumatol* 1985;**14**(1):1–7.
23 Ostensen M, Skavdal K, Myklebust G, Tomassen Y, Aarbakke J. Excretion of gold into human breast milk. *Eur J Clin Pharmacol* 1986;**31**(2):251–2.
24 Temprano KK, Bandlamudi R, Moore TL. Antirheumatic drugs in pregnancy and lactation. *Semin Arthritis Rheum* 2005;**35**(2):112–21.
25 Chakravarty EF, Sanchez-Yamamoto D, Bush TM. The use of disease modifying antirheumatic drugs in women with rheumatoid arthritis of childbearing age: a survey of practice patterns and pregnancy outcomes. *J Rheumatol* 2003;**30**(2):241–6.
26 Miehle W. Current aspects of D-penicillamine and pregnancy. *Z Rheumatol* 1988;**47**(Suppl 1):20–3.
27 Scheinberg IH, Sternlieb I. Pregnancy in penicillamine-treated patients with Wilson's disease. *N Engl J Med* 1975;**293**(25):1300–2.
28 Walshe JM. Pregnancy in Wilson's disease. *Q J Med* 1977;**46**(181):73–83.
29 Schroder H, Fogh K. Methotrexate and its polyglutamate derivatives in erythrocytes during and after weekly low-dose oral methotrexate

therapy of children with acute lymphoblastic leukemia. *Cancer Chemother Pharmacol* 1988;**21**(2):145–9.

30 Hausknecht RU. Methotrexate and misoprostol to terminate early pregnancy. *N Engl J Med* 1995;**333**(9):537–40.

31 Schleuning M, Clemm C. Chromosomal aberrations in a newborn whose mother received cytotoxic treatment during pregnancy. *N Engl J Med* 1987;**317**(26):1666–7.

32 Johns DG, Rutherford LD, Leighton PC, Vogel CL. Secretion of methotrexate into human milk. *Am J Obstet Gynecol* 1972;**112**(7):978–80.

33 Armenti VT, Ahlswede KM, Ahlswede BA, Jarrell BE, Moritz MJ, Burke JF. National transplantation pregnancy registry – outcomes of 154 pregnancies in cyclosporine-treated female kidney transplant recipients. *Transplantation* 1994;**57**(4):502–6.

34 Hussein MM, Mooij JM, Roujouleh H. Cyclosporine in the treatment of lupus nephritis including two patients treated during pregnancy. *Clin Nephrol* 1993;**40**(3):160–3.

35 Moretti M, Sgro M, Johnson D, Sauve R, Woolgar M. Cyclosporin excretion into breast milk. *Transplantation* 2003;**7**:3144–6.

36 Polifka JE, Friedman JM. Teratogen update: azathioprine and 6-mercaptopurine. *Teratology* 2002;**65**(5):240–61.

37 Scott JR. Fetal growth retardation associated with maternal administration of immunosuppressive drugs. *Am J Obstet Gynecol* 1977;**128**(6):668–76.

38 Cote CJ, Meuwissen HJ, Pickering RJ. Effects on the neonate of prednisone and azathioprine administered to the mother during pregnancy. *J Pediatr* 1974;**85**(3):324–8.

39 Davison JM, Dellagrammatikas H, Parkin JM. Maternal azathioprine therapy and depressed haemopoiesis in the babies of renal allograft patients. *Br J Obstet Gynaecol* 1985;**92**(3):233–9.

40 Hayslett JP, Lynn RI. Effect of pregnancy in patients with lupus nephropathy. *Kidney Int* 1980;**18**(2):207–20.

41 Meehan RT, Dorsey JK. Pregnancy among patients with systemic lupus erythematosus receiving immunosuppressive therapy. *J Rheumatol* 1987;**14**(2):252–8.

42 Bermas BL, Hill JA. Effects of immunosuppressive drugs during pregnancy. *Arthritis Rheum* 1995;**38**(12):1722–32.

43 Lockshin MD. Fertility in systemic lupus erythematosus. In Tsokos G, Gordon C, Smolen J (eds), *Systemic Lupus Erythematosus: A Companion to Rheumatology*, 1st edition. Philadelphia: Mosby Elsevier; 2007:460–5.

44 Kirshon B, Wasserstrum N, Willis R, Herman GE, McCabe ER. Teratogenic effects of first-trimester cyclophosphamide therapy. *Obstet Gynecol* 1988;**72**(3 Pt 2):462–4.

45 Gershenson DM. Menstrual and reproductive function after treatment with combination chemotherapy for malignant ovarian germ cell tumors. *J Clin Oncol* 1988;**6**(2):270–5.

46 Clowse ME, Magder L, Petri M. Cyclophosphamide for lupus during pregnancy. *Lupus* 2005;**14**(8):593–7.
47 Wiernik PH, Duncan JH. Cyclophosphamide in human milk. *Lancet* 1971;**1**(7705):912.
48 Carter JD, Valeriano J, Vasey FB. Tumor necrosis factor-alpha inhibition and VATER association: a causal relationship. *J Rheumatol* 2006;**33**(5):1014–7.

CHAPTER 8

Psychotropic drugs in pregnancy

Neelam Sisodia

Introduction

Women taking psychotropic drugs in pregnancy fall into two groups: those who are actively being treated for a pre-existing psychiatric disorder and those who develop symptoms of psychiatric disorder during the course of their pregnancy. Of the latter group, some will have a history of psychiatric disorder, and their symptoms signify relapse of the pre-existing condition and the rest will be experiencing an illness for the first time.

The prevalence of psychiatric disorder during pregnancy is the same as in non-childbearing women of the same age. Between 15 and 20% of all pregnant women will have a mental health problem [1], ranging from mild to moderate illnesses such as generalised anxiety, mild depression, obsessional compulsive disorder and anxiety with panic/phobic symptoms to severe illnesses such as moderate to severe depression, bipolar affective disorder and schizophrenia.

The National Institute for Health and Clinical Excellence (NICE) guideline on antenatal and postnatal mental health [2] recommends that wherever possible, psychosocial interventions and psychological therapies (supportive psychotherapy, cognitive behavioural therapy and interpersonal therapy) should be first-line treatment for mild to moderate conditions. The threshold for using psychotropic medication should be relatively high and it should be prescribed only if a psychological approach alone does not alleviate symptoms.

Prescribing in Pregnancy, 4th edition. Edited by Peter Rubin and Margaret Ramsay,
 ISBN: 978-1-4051-4712-5.

Severe illnesses, in which psychotic symptoms may play a part, are more likely to severely disrupt a woman's capacity to care for herself during pregnancy and her baby after delivery, if untreated. Whilst psychological approaches continue to play a positive role in treatment of these conditions, medication plays a more important role than in minor disorders, and the threshold for its use is lower. As all women of childbearing age may potentially become pregnant, these women should, as part of their treatment plan, be informed of the importance of using adequate contraception to avoid pregnancy whilst taking drugs that may potentially harm the fetus, at the same time also being given information about the potential adverse effects on the fetus/newborn of untreated maternal psychiatric disorder. Wherever possible, these women should be helped to plan pregnancy during a period of remission in illness, so that they are able to conceive free of psychotropic medication. Ideally they should be managed without psychotropic medication for the whole of the first trimester. If this is not possible, then the aim should be to use the lowest dose of medication that gives adequate symptom control.

The aim of initiating or continuing treatment of significant and enduring mental illnesses with psychotropic medication during pregnancy is to alleviate suffering during this time but also to prevent deterioration/relapse postpartum. A detailed discussion of psychiatric disorder in pregnancy and postpartum is beyond the scope of this chapter. However, it should be noted that despite the recommendations and findings of the previous enquiry, the last Confidential Enquiry into Maternal and Child Health [3] found that psychiatric causes of death are the second leading indirect cause of maternal death in the UK. If all maternal deaths, including those ascertained by the Office of National Statistics Linkage Study are included, then suicide emerges as the leading cause of maternal death, accounting for 15%, and psychiatric conditions contribute to 25% of all maternal deaths.

Every effort should therefore be made during the early antenatal period to identify women at significant risk of developing a serious psychiatric disorder during pregnancy or postpartum [4], because of a pre-existing condition, new onset illness or a strong family history of serious illness. Care can then be coordinated appropriately between primary care medical and midwifery practitioners and secondary level general adult psychiatric and obstetric services, liaising wherever possible with subspecialists in perinatal psychiatry, in case of need for specialist advice about medication, community outreach services or inpatient admission to a psychiatric Mother and Baby facility [5].

Whilst the ideal is that women should plan conception at a time when they are psychologically well and not taking psychotropic medication, in reality approximately 50% of pregnancies are unplanned at the point of conception. Approximately 33% [6,7] of women have been shown to be taking prescribed medication during the first trimester of pregnancy and a significant proportion of these are taking psychotropic preparations. The natural inclination of most women in this day and age is to discontinue treatment immediately on discovering a pregnancy, for fear of the adverse consequences of medication on the developing fetus. However, doctors and other health professionals caring for these women should advise caution in discontinuing medication immediately.

Women suffering from a mild to moderate psychiatric disorder who become pregnant whilst taking antidepressant preparations prescribed in primary care should be advised to withdraw from medication gradually, as abrupt discontinuation of treatment may cause unpleasant withdrawal symptoms, adding to any distress and anxiety about fetal exposure to a potential teratogen.

In the case of women receiving treatment for a severe psychiatric disorder, a thorough evaluation needs to be made of the risks versus the benefits. There is potential risk to the fetus of adverse effects of psychotropic medication at various stages throughout pregnancy, and not just at the stage of organogenesis, which has usually been completed by the time an accidental pregnancy is discovered. There is also risk to the fetus, however, if the mother has a relapse of a serious mental illness that compromises obstetric and psychiatric care and the safety of mother and fetus. If this is a significant risk, then it will be of greater benefit for a woman to continue treatment, even if the psychotropic preparation has to be changed to allow for maximal safety in pregnancy. A woman conceiving accidentally whilst taking psychotropic medication with potential for causing harm to the fetus should have early access to detailed ultrasound scanning to determine the effects of exposure so that a wanted pregnancy is not unnecessarily terminated.

As virtually all psychotropic drugs cross the placenta, any such preparation administered to a pregnant woman will reach the embryo and fetus. The timing of exposure to psychotropic drugs is of particular importance to the development of the central nervous and cardiovascular systems (development of central nervous system begins between day 16 and 18 and the neural tube closes by day 30, two weeks after a missed period; the various structures within the heart are formed between day 22 and 35, five weeks after the last period). As the central nervous system continues to develop throughout fetal life and early infancy, its structural and functional development remains vulnerable to adverse effects from psychotropic medication (and any other potentially noxious substances) until the end of pregnancy and beyond [8–10].

General Principles

- Psychosocial interventions and psychological therapies should be the first-line approach to mild to moderate (non-psychotic) psychiatric disorder.
- Severe psychiatric disorders, especially those accompanied by psychotic symptoms, require robust management as the consequences of untreated severe psychiatric disorder have great adverse consequences for mother and fetus/infant.
- If medication is felt to be necessary in addition to psychological treatment, involve the pregnant woman in the discussion to treat.
- The evidence base is changing continuously. In general, there is much more information available about older preparations, both in terms of potential adverse effects and benefits, and so it is best to avoid newer drugs.
- Physiological and pharmacokinetics changes occurring in pregnancy affect drug metabolism and therefore the doses of medication may need to be adjusted.
- Use the lowest effective dose, dividing it through the day if practicable with patient compliance.
- Avoid using more than one preparation wherever possible.
- Consider tapering the doses of medication towards the end of pregnancy, discontinuing wherever possible (i.e., as long as the risk of deterioration in the pregnant woman's mental state is not greater than the risk of adverse effects in the neonate) by 36–38 wk of gestation.

Tricyclic antidepressants

Imipramine is the prototype tricyclic antidepressant (TCA). Other drugs in this group include amitriptyline, clomipramine, dosulepin, dothiepin, lofepramine, trimipramine, desipramine and nortriptyline.

TCAs have been in use for over 40 years. There is no evidence of an association between treatment with TCAs and an increased incidence of birth defects or other adverse pregnancy outcome (although a few case reports exist from the 1970s to 1980s, associating tricyclic antidepressants with congenital limb and heart malformations, polydactyly and hypospadias) [11]. Care must still be taken towards the end of pregnancy, however, as short-lived neonatal withdrawal symptoms such as jitteriness, hyperexcitability, myoclonus, convulsions and sucking problems have been reported very occasionally, particularly in premature or small-for-dates infants. To date, there is no indication that use of TCAs in pregnancy causes adverse effects on children in terms of neurodevelopment such as global IQ, language and behaviour (in contrast to evidence available linking untreated severe depression in the mother with poor cognitive development and behavioural disorder in children, persistent to the age of 11 yr, especially in male children).

TCAs have fallen out of favour in recent years, both in primary care and general adult psychiatry because of the potential for acute poisoning (especially cardiotoxicity) when used to self-harm and for possible intolerance of anticholinergic side effects. However, if a thorough assessment of potential for self-harm is undertaken, medication supplied in small quantities and the dose titrated slowly, there is no reason why TCAs should not be used where significant and disabling depressive symptoms exist.

Imipramine and amitriptyline are in fact at present considered to be the drugs of choice when treating moderate to severe depression during pregnancy [12] and can be used to control severe and disabling symptoms of anxiety and panic that have not been ameliorated by psychological interventions. TCAs also have the advantage of being excreted in low concentrations in breast milk and there is no evidence to suggest that they cause harm to the neonate/infant. Treatment with TCAs can therefore be reinstated following delivery in breastfeeding mothers.

Selective serotonin/noradrenaline reuptake inhibitor antidepressants

The use of selective serotonin reuptake inhibitor antidepressants (SSRIs) such as citalopram, fluoxetine, fluvoxamine, paroxetine and sertraline has increased over the last decade, especially as first-line drug treatment for mild to moderate depression. It has been much emphasised that SSRIs are better tolerated than TCAs and are safer in overdose.

Previously considered to be relatively safe in pregnancy and breastfeeding, the SSRIs are an example of how the evidence base may change over time for new drugs. In recent years there have been a number of studies and case reports associating SSRIs and venlafaxine with a variety of neonatal complications such as prematurity, low birth weight, neonatal respiratory and neurobehavioural difficulties and increased admission to neonatal units. Also, there has been an association with higher incidence of three or more minor congenital anomalies and neonatal withdrawal symptoms with the use of fluoxetine. The likelihood of persistent pulmonary hypertension of the newborn in infants exposed to SSRIs in late pregnancy (after 20 wk of gestation) is now thought to be increased up to sixfold [13]. Paroxetine has been associated with ventricular septal defects and atrial septal defects [14], with the risk being increased approximately twofold compared to that in the general population. It remains to be seen whether this is a class effect of SSRIs or is specific to paroxetine, but at present the NICE guideline on antenatal and postnatal mental health does not recommend paroxetine in pregnancy.

There is also increasing evidence that SSRIs and venlafaxine can be associated with troublesome neonatal withdrawal symptoms [15], noted to be most severe with paroxetine. Though SSRIs are not absolutely contraindicated in pregnancy, exposed neonates may need careful monitoring in a neonatal unit as the problems (abnormal movements, hypo/hypertonia, insomnia and dyspnoea) can persist for up to 5 days.

SSRIs have been associated with bleeding disorders in adults, and there are case reports involving newborns. Infants exposed to fluoxetine prenatally may have an increased haemorrhagic tendency. SSRIs continue to be used at present in breastfeeding women but some preparations such as fluoxetine and citalopram have been reported to cause irritability and poor-feeding in infants, especially those who are premature or have low birth weight. Sertraline is at present associated with least problems in breastfeeding.

Key point

- Imipramine and amitriptyline should be considered as first-line choice when antidepressants are required in pregnancy

Mood-stabilising drugs

Mood-stabilising drugs such as lithium and the anti-epileptic drugs carbamazepine, sodium valproate and lamotrigine may be used by psychiatrists in the treatment of acute mania, as maintenance treatment for bipolar affective disorder and as augmentation in the treatment of chronic resistant depression. All mood-stabilising drugs are potentially teratogenic and fetotoxic, and the adverse effects of anti-epileptic drugs are as applicable when used in psychiatric disorder as they are when used in women with epilepsy.

Women with bipolar affective disorder particularly are likely to use a mood-stabiliser preparation for a substantial proportion of their reproductive life. It is therefore important that they are made aware of the risks involved in childbearing, both from the treatments used and from their discontinuation. The NICE guideline on antenatal and postnatal mental health recommends that if a woman with bipolar affective disorder is planning pregnancy or is already pregnant, a low dose of an antipsychotic drug is preferable to a mood-stabilising agent both for the acute treatment of mania and as prophylaxis in those whose mental state is stable. Anti-epileptic drugs are dealt with in Chapter 9.

Lithium

Lithium has long been known to be associated with congenital malformations of the heart, in particular Ebstein's anomaly, involving abnormalities of the tricuspid valve. However, in recent years, it has been established that the risk of Ebstein's anomaly in exposed pregnancies is not as high as previously estimated. The current information available suggests that the increased incidence of Ebstein's anomaly is between 1:1000 and 1:2000, against a background incidence of 1:200,000. Although the estimated risk of Ebstein's anomaly in lithium-exposed infants is 10–20 times higher than expected, the absolute risk is small (0.05–1.00%). Analysis of combined data from several studies indicates that the overall risk of congenital heart disease varies from 0.9 to 12.0% in lithium-exposed pregnancies compared with 0.5–1.0% in the general population [16].

Other risks associated with lithium have not been quantified, but there have been case reports of polyhydramnios after fetal polyuria, neonatal diabetes insipidus, arrhythmias, jaundice and hypothyroidism. Because of rapidly changing maternal plasma volume around the time of delivery, serum lithium levels may increase markedly, causing both maternal and neonatal toxicity. A 'floppy infant' syndrome has been described in this context, characterised by lethargy, hypotonia, cyanosis, tachypnoea, tachycardia and poor sucking.

Women accidentally conceiving on lithium should not abruptly discontinue treatment as there is a significant risk of relapse of their illness. An early, detailed ultrasound scan will clarify whether or not the exposed fetus has a congenital heart defect, allowing the pregnant woman to make an informed decision about continuing pregnancy.

The various sources reviewed [17–19] suggest that lithium is the drug of choice when a mood stabiliser is required in pregnancy. However, for many women it may not be acceptable that in addition to the possibility of congenital cardiac malformations from exposure in early pregnancy, there may be fetotoxic effects with continued lithium use in later pregnancy. These individuals may choose therefore not to use lithium and instead be monitored closely for early signs of relapse, commencing a small dose of a typical antipsychotic such as haloperidol or trifluoperazine as soon as necessary.

Whether lithium is used in pregnancy will very much depend on a case-by-case consideration of the risks and benefits, and any particular woman's past history of remission/relapse and response to treatment. The woman should be closely involved in the decision made.

Key points

Lithium use in pregnancy

- The pregnancy should be confirmed as early as possible and an ultrasound scan be arranged to establish gestation.
- An urgent referral to a specialist in fetomaternal medicine should be made.
- Lithium should not be stopped abruptly because of high risk of relapse.
- If a woman has been previously well for 2 yr or more, lithium may be slowly withdrawn during pregnancy by 200 mg every 4 wk.
- If the woman is judged to be at high risk of relapse if the lithium is withdrawn, the continuation of lithium in pregnancy may be necessary. Lithium levels should be monitored monthly until 28 wk of gestation and weekly thereafter.

(Continued)

(*Continued*)

- Urea and electrolytes and thyroid function should be regularly monitored.
- A further detailed ultrasound scan will be necessary to exclude major congenital cardiac abnormalities even if the lithium has been discontinued shortly before or after conception.
- Lithium should be tapered and withdrawn by 38 wk of gestation wherever clinically possible.
- If for any reason, for example, deterioration in a woman's mental state or preterm delivery, a woman is still taking lithium at the onset of labour, lithium levels will need to be monitored during labour and in the immediate postpartum period because of the dangers of a sudden rise in maternal serum levels.
- Lithium should be reinstated at 400 mg daily on day 1 postpartum, gradually increasing to the pre-pregnancy dose over 14 days, with initial weekly monitoring of serum levels whilst ensuring adequate hydration.
- Lithium is excreted in significant concentrations in breast milk and therefore not recommended in breastfeeding mothers (an antipsychotic drug may be offered instead).

Antipsychotic drugs

Antipsychotic drugs are used in the management of acute and chronic psychiatric disorders such as bipolar affective disorder (depressive psychosis, hypomania, mania) and schizophrenia and schizophrenia-like illnesses. Individuals in remission may continue to take oral or depot preparations of antipsychotic drugs. Though some of the older 'typical' antipsychotic drugs, which work by blocking dopamine receptors, could potentially reduce fertility by increasing serum prolactin levels, the newer 'atypical' antipsychotic drugs do not tend to have this effect (risperidone and amisulpiride excepted). Women taking antipsychotic preparations may therefore become pregnant and may wish to continue with pregnancy. The adverse effects of an acute or chronic psychotic illness in the mother will generally outweigh the risks to the fetus of antipsychotic medication and it is important to treat psychotic illnesses robustly.

Typical antipsychotic drugs

Data on the use of phenothiazines (chlorpromazine, trifluoperazine and fluphenazine) in pregnancy is based on studies of hyperemesis gravidarum. As smaller doses of medication are used for this condition than in psychotic illnesses, this should be borne in mind when assessing the risks versus the benefits. There have been case reports of congenital malformations such as microcephaly, syndactyly and cardiac defects associated with phenothiazine use, but larger studies have failed to demonstrate a significant risk. There is little evidence of teratogenicity linked to the use of haloperidol, a typical antipsychotic of the butyrophenone group.

In clinical practice, if a degree of sedation is required in an acute psychotic illness, then chlorpromazine can be used in divided doses. Trifluoperazine and haloperidol are the drugs of choice otherwise. It is best practice to prescribe antipsychotics as oral preparations in pregnancy to allow greater flexibility in dose adjustment. The NICE guideline on antenatal and postnatal mental health does not recommend the routine use of depot antipsychotic preparations in pregnancy as extrapyramidal side effects can occur in the neonate/infant several months after administration. Fluphenazine is in any case the only antipsychotic preparation available as depot in the UK for which data on use during pregnancy is available.

Phenothiazines and haloperidol may cause withdrawal symptoms or transient extrapyramidal symptoms in the neonate and therefore wherever possible, treatment should be withdrawn by 36–38 weeks of gestation.

Atypical antipsychotic drugs

The newer 'atypical' antipsychotic drugs have been used with increasing frequency over the last decade as they are said to be better tolerated in terms of sedation and extrapyramidal side effects. As dopamine receptor blockade is weaker in this group of drugs, prolactin levels tend not to be raised and therefore fertility is not decreased. Pregnancy may occur at times of changing over from a typical to an atypical antipsychotic preparation.

The database for the use and effects of atypical antipsychotic drugs is small at present. A number of case reports exist, describing the diverse outcomes of pregnancies exposed to clozapine. These include maternal hyperglycaemia and gestational diabetes as well as fetal and neonatal problems (floppy infant syndrome, seizures and unspecified malformations). Clozapine cannot be recommended in pregnancy at present, associated as it is with agranulocytosis in adult patients. Case reports on the use of olanzapine in pregnancy do not at present link it with any specific congenital abnormality, but gestational diabetes, fetal macrosomia, neonatal cardiomegaly, jaundice and convulsions have been described [20]. Little is known about the use of risperidone and quetiapine in pregnancy at present.

Key points

- The antipsychotics of choice in pregnancy are trifluoperazine and haloperidol.
- Use oral preparations, in the lowest dose possible (this will also reduce the risk of extrapyramidal side effects as antimuscarinic drugs are not recommended in pregnancy).
- Taper the dose and discontinue treatment between 36 and 38 wk of gestation wherever clinically possible.
- Observe neonates for adverse effects.
- Trifluoperazine and haloperidol may be used in breastfeeding.

References

1 Oates M. Psychiatric disorders in pregnancy and the post-partum period. In: Greer I, Nelson-Piercy C and Walters B (eds.), *Maternal Medicine: Medical Problems in Pregnancy*. New York: Churchill-Livingstone; 2007:295–308.

2 National Institute for Health and Clinical Excellence. *Antenatal and Postnatal Mental Health: Clinical Management and Service Guidance*. NICE Guideline Number 45; 2007.

3 Oates M for CEMACH. Deaths from psychiatric causes. In: *Why Mothers Die 2000–2002*, Sixth Report of the Confidential Enquiries into Maternal Deaths in the United Kingdom. London: Royal College of Obstericians and Gynaecologists; 2004:152–73.

4 Cantwell R, Oates M. Screening in pregnancy for serious risk of postnatal mental illness. In: O'Keane V, Marsh M, Senevratne G (eds.), *Psychiatric Disorders in Pregnancy*. London and New York: Taylor & Francis Group; 2006:5–20.

5 Royal College of Psychiatrists Council. *Perinatal Maternal Mental Health Services*, Report CR88. London: Royal College of Psychiatrists; 2000.

6 Rubin P. Drug treatment in pregnancy. *BMJ* 1998;**317**:1503–6.

7 Wilton LV, Pearce GL, Martin RM, Mackay FJ and Mann RD. The outcomes of pregnancy in women exposed to newly marketed drugs in general practice in England. *Br J Obstet Gynaecol* 1998;**105**:882–9.

8 McElhatton P. Teratogenicity and psychotropic drug use in pregnancy. In: O'Keane V, Marsh M, Senevratne G (eds.), *Psychiatric Disorders in Pregnancy.* London and New York: Taylor & Francis Group; 2006:223–46.
9 Wieck A. Management of psychosis before, during and after pregnancy. In: O'Keane V, Marsh M, Senevratne G (eds.), *Psychiatric Disorders in Pregnancy.* London and New York: Taylor & Francis Group; 2006:107–24.
10 Sanz E, De-las-Cuevas C, Kiuru A, Bate A and Edwards R. Selective serotonin-reuptake inhibitors in pregnant women and neonatal withdrawal syndrome: a database analysis. *Lancet* 2005;**365**:482–7.
11 Garbis H, McElhatton P. Psychotropic, sedative-hypnotic and Parkinson drugs. In: Schaefer C (ed.), *Drugs in Pregnancy and Lactation.* Amsterdam: Elsevier Science; 2001:182–91.
12 The National Teratology Information Service (NTIS). Treatment of depression in pregnancy. Monograph, 2005.
13 Chambers CD, Hernandez-Diaz S, Van Marter LJ, Werler MM, Louik C, Jones KL and Mitchell AA. Selective serotonin-reuptake inhibitors and risk of persistent pulmonary hypertension of the newborn. *N Engl J Med* 2006;**354**:579–87.
14 The National Teratology Information Service (NTIS). Use of Paroxetine in pregnancy. Monograph, 2005.
15 Ferreira E, Carcellar AM, Agogue C, Martin BZ, St-Andre M, Francoeur D and Berard A. Effects of selective serotonin-reuptake inhibitors and venlafaxine during pregnancy in term and pre-term neonates. *Pediatrics* 2007;**119**:52–9.
16 Viguera AC, Cohen LS, Baldessarini RJ and Nonacs R. Managing bipolar disorder during pregnancy: weighing the risks and benefits. *Can J Psych* 2002;**47**(5):426–36.
17 Llewelyn A, Stowe ZN, Strader JRJ. The use of lithium and management of women with bipolar disorder during pregnancy and lactation [review]. *J Clin Psychiat* 1998;**59**(Suppl 6):57–64.
18 Garbis H and McElhatton P. Psychotropic, sedative-hypnotic and Parkinson drugs. In: Schaefer C (ed.) *Drugs in pregnancy and lactation.* Amsterdam: Elsevier Science; 2001:182–91.
19 McElhatton P. Teratogenicity and psychotropic drug use in pregnancy. In: O'Keane V, Marsh M and Senevratne G (eds.) *Psychiatric disorders in pregnancy.* London and New York: Taylor & Francis Group; 2006:223–46.
20 The National Teratology Information Service (NTIS). Minipreg summaries on clozapine, olanzapine, quetiapine and risperidone 2002.

CHAPTER 9

Managing epilepsy and anti-epileptic drugs during pregnancy

Michael F. O'Donoghue, Christine P. Hayes

Introduction

Women with epilepsy comprise 6/1000 pregnancies [1]. Most women taking anti-epileptic drugs (AEDs) during pregnancy give birth to healthy babies that subsequently develop normally. Nevertheless, many pregnant women with epilepsy fear that AEDs, or seizures, may harm the developing infant. As a result some women stop treatment of their own accord [1,2]. Subsequent seizure relapse will have repercussions on occupation and the possession of a driving licence. These considerations are a worry for women with epilepsy and their doctors. The relevant literature is now very large and, in part, conflicting. Much of it is affected by methodological problems. For some topics there is insufficient evidence to guide decision making. We provide a concise review of the facts and provide practical advice. Our priorities are the safety of the mother and the developing infant and to anticipate problems by providing optimum advice before conception. A number of recent reviews provide further reading [3–6].

The evidence concerning epilepsy and pregnancy

Anti-epileptic drugs and the developing infant

It is not fully understood why AEDs can be teratogenic. An orthodox view holds that the period of risk is the first trimester [7].

Prescribing in Pregnancy, 4th edition. Edited by Peter Rubin and Margaret Ramsay,
 ISBN: 978-1-4051-4712-5.

However, the older literature has mostly focused on structural abnormalities visible at birth and has often not followed children long enough to detect effects on cognition and behaviour. Brain development occurs in a complex and protracted sequence. Neuronal cell production continues until the fifth month (and in some regions beyond this time), migration into the sixth month and cortical differentiation and myelination beyond birth [8–10]. Thus, there may be a series of critical periods throughout pregnancy during which, theoretically, drugs could disrupt development, with later effects being functional rather than structural [11]. More recent research addresses the cognitive and behavioural consequences of gestational AED exposure, and some studies give cause for concern.

Mechanisms of teratogenesis

There are several possible mechanisms of teratogenesis by AEDs [12]. An early theory stated that it arose as a result of altered folate metabolism. Another hypothesis links embryonic bradycardia (caused by AEDs) with ischaemia-evoked malformations [13]. A further idea is that AEDs are metabolised to highly reactive intermediates that interact harmfully with cellular macromolecules (e.g., DNA) [12]. Pharmacogenetic factors (in the embryo and the mother) determine the concentration of these intermediates. Infants of mothers that metabolise these intermediates poorly may be at higher risk. In humans there is evidence that this applies to phenytoin and valproate [14,15]. Embryonic metabolism may, possibly, also be able to activate AEDs to molecules that damage DNA and interfere with signalling [12]. Valproate may have specific mechanisms of teratogenesis related to altered gene expression during development [16,17]. In animal models, genetic factors determine susceptibility to teratogenesis [18]. In humans it has been reported that dizygotic twins can be discordant for the harmful effects of in utero exposure to phenytoin, or valproate, yet other women have pregnancies repeatedly affected by malformations [19–21]. This evidence underscores the importance of genetic factors in teratogenesis.

Folate

Folate is essential to DNA synthesis and appropriate gene expression during embryonic development. Folate requires a dietary source as it cannot be synthesized in the body. Low serum folate levels in the general population are linked to neural tube defects (NTDs), and supplementation during pregnancy prevents the first occurrence and recurrence in high-risk cases [22–24]. Phenytoin, phenobarbitone and carbamazepine cause low serum folate levels [25–27]. Folate antagonists taken in pregnancy are associated with cardiac, urogenital and neural tube defects [28,29]. Low serum folate levels in pregnant women taking AEDs are associated with an increased malformation rate [25,26,30]. Mutations in maternal, but not paternal, enzymes involved in folate metabolism place some infants at a higher risk of fetal anticonvulsant syndrome [31]. It is unclear to what extent folate supplementation protects against different malformations. It is also unknown whether any effect extends to all AEDs. There is conflicting evidence whether folate can prevent valproate-induced NTDs in animals [32–34]. Reports of infants with NTDs whose mothers took adequate folate imply the protection is incomplete [19,35,36]. Nevertheless, as the neural tube closes by the end of the fourth week of pregnancy, it is vital that folate is taken before conception. A theoretical concern that folate could worsen epilepsy control has not been borne out in practice [37].

Types of malformations associated with anti-epileptic drugs

AEDs taken during pregnancy have been associated with major malformations (MM, defined as a physical defect causing major functional disturbance and requiring intervention), minor anomalies (defined as deviations from normal morphology not requiring intervention), growth retardation and neurodevelopmental problems [12,20]. The commonest MM are NTDs (spina bifida and hydrocephalus), cardiac malformations, hypospadias, palatal and lip clefts, and skeletal deformities. The first generation of drugs (phenobarbitone and phenytoin) were most closely associated with heart, facial and digital defects (the latter especially with phenytoin) [12,38]. The next generation of drugs (carbamazepine and valproate) caused NTDs and hypospadias [12,39–42]. The risk of spina bifida with valproate is about 2%, and is usually a severe open lumbosacral defect with hydrocephalus [39]. The risk of spina bifida with carbamazepine is about 1% [43]. Midfacial and limb anomalies have been associated with particular AEDs, or AEDs collectively, and have been called the 'fetal anticonvulsant syndrome'. These anomalies include (a) wide-spaced eyes, depressed nasal bridge, low-set ears and distal digital hypoplasia (phenytoin and carbamazepine), and (b) high forehead, depressed nasal bridge, upturned nose, deficient inner eyebrow, long philtrum, thin upper lip and ophthalmologic problems (valproate) [44,45]. Infants with the fetal valproate syndrome may also have musculoskeletal, cardiovascular, urogenital or pulmonary malformations in varying proportions [46]. Further features of the fetal phenytoin syndrome include microcephaly, growth deficiency, with or without craniofacial and cardiac malformation [47]. Some have argued that there is a discernable carbamazepine facies too [48]. There is concern that midface anomalies correlate with decreased intelligence [49,50]. The children of women with epilepsy not taking AEDs may have some facial features of the syndrome (e.g., epicanthal folds) but not the full syndrome [48,51].

The risk of major malformations

The risks of MM have been analysed in many retrospective studies and more recently in prospective registry studies. The outcomes are highly dependent on the method of ascertainment and case definition, making study comparisons difficult. Nevertheless, reviews of studies before the 1990s have suggested a two- to threefold increase of MM over the general population in those on AEDs [52]. Given the changes in AED prescribing practice, it is important to review the outcome of more recent studies (Table 9.1). The rate of MM in the general (non-epileptic) population from older studies was 3–4% [38]. In recent studies, general population MM rates were 1.5% [41], 1.8% [55], 2.3% [61] and 2.3% [53]. The rates in women with epilepsy who did not take AEDs were 0.8% [30], 2.7% [61], 2.8% [58], 3.1% [54] and 3.5% [59]. A meta-analysis concluded that the risk of malformations in women with epilepsy and not on medication was no different from the general population [62].

Most studies confirm the increased risk of MM in infants to exposed AEDs over the general population. The majority of studies confirm an approximate doubling of risk of polytherapy over monotherapy [30,41,54–56,59]. The rates for monotherapy with carbamazepine, phenytoin and lamotrigine do not differ significantly from each other except for one study in which the rate for phenytoin was unusually low [41]. In one study the risk for carbamazepine monotherapy was not significantly greater than control [58]. A meta-analysis of studies on carbamazepine with

Table 9.1 Major malformation rate (%) in infants exposed to AED monotherapy (number of infants exposed) in recent large studies

Study author (Date)	All monotherapy	Carbamazepine	Valproate	Phenytoin	Lamotrigine
Canger (1999) [53]	5.7 (313)	6.2 (113)	13.6 (44)	0.0	—
Kaneko (1999) [54]	7.8 (500)	5.7 (158)	11.1 (81)	9.1 (132)	
Samren (1999) [41]	3.3 (899)	3.7 (376)	5.7 (158)	0.6 (151)	
Holmes (2001) [55]	4.5 (223)	5.2 (58)	—	3.4 (87)	
Kaaja (2003) [30]	3.2 (594)	2.8 (363)	6.6 (61)	2.4 (124)	
Wide (2004) [56]	5.4 (1256)	4.0 (703)	9.7 (268)	6.8 (103)	4.4 (90)
Wyszynski (2004) [36]	—	—	10.7 (149)	—	—
Cunnington (2005) [57]	—	—	—	—	2.9 (414)
Artama (2005) [58]	4.2 (1231)	2.7 (805)	10.6 (263)	—	
Morrow (2006) [59]	3.7 (2468)	2.2 (900)	6.2 (715)	3.7 (82)	3.2 (647)
Holmes (2006) [60]					2.7 (564)

1255 exposed subjects, which did not include UK registry data, found a monotherapy malformation rate of 5.2% [61]. The UK registry reported a 2.2% MM rate in 900 carbamazepine exposures [59]. Several studies report that the MM rate for valproate exceeds other drugs by two- to threefold [36,56,58,59,63]. The risk increases appreciably if the valproate dose exceeds 800–1000 mg [36,41,54,56,58,59,64,65]. Studies have pointed to high rates in barbiturate exposures: phenobarbitone (6.5%) [66] and primidone (14%) [54]. Lamotrigine is gaining ground as monotherapy in both partial and generalized epilepsies. The manufacturer's registry observed an MM rate of 2.9% (CI, 1.6–5.1) in 414 exposures [57]. The UK registry found an MM rate of 3.2% (95% CI, 2.1–4.9) in 647 monotherapy exposures [59]. There was a clear dose-response effect for lamotrigine. The MM rate with doses up to 200 mg was 1.7%, but with doses above 200 mg it was 5.4%, which was no different to valproate exposures up to 1000 mg (5.1%). The North American registry recently reported a 2.7% MM rate for 564 lamotrigine exposures compared to 1.6% unexposed [60]. An increased risk of oral clefts following exposure to lamotrigine has been reported. In the North American registry there were 5 oral clefts among 564 exposed infants [60]. In five other registries there were 4 clefts in 1623 lamotrigine exposures [60]. Further work is required to quantify the risk.

There is insufficient information to decide if any particular polytherapy regime is less risky. Data from the UK registry found no MM in 118 combined carbamazepine and lamotrigine exposures. Combinations of valproate and carbamazepine have an MM rate of about 10% [40,58,59]. Combinations of valproate with lamotrigine have an MM rate of 9–12% [57,59]. Whether benzodiazepines are associated with MM is disputed. A meta-analysis of studies in 1997 concluded that cohort studies revealed no association but case-control studies showed an odds ratio for MM of 3 [67]. A more recent study found an increased MM risk, though the authors considered it was due to recall bias [68]. Reviews have concluded that there is no clear evidence of an increased MM rate [69,70]. One study found cases of MM associated with ethosuximide use [40]; another observed none in 12 monotherapy exposures [59]. There is a large literature on limb and brain malformations in rodents associated with acetazolamide [71], but there is almost no information about humans except a single case with an MM [41].

The risk with new anti-epileptic drugs

There is much less information about new AEDs. Exposures to oxcarbazepine were associated with one MM each in 99 [58] and 55 exposures [72]. In the UK registry, topiramate monotherapy was associated with two MM in 28 exposures, gabapentin one in 31 and levetiracetam none in 25 [59]. Given the absence of clinical data, knowledge of the effects in animals is relevant. A review of the animal data found oxcarbazepine, tiagabine (high dose), topiramate (low doses) and zonisamide to be definitely teratogenic [6]. Levetiracetam at high doses caused skeletal abnormalities and growth retardation, but no gross malformations. No developmental toxicity was noted at clinically relevant doses in vigabatrin, gabapentin or pregabalin.

The effect of seizures on fetal development

The literature on the effect of seizures on fetal development is sparse. Case reports document the effect of tonic-clonic, eclamptic or complex partial seizures on fetal heart rate [73–77]. Decelerations of fetal heart rate were seen, though this was not associated with a poor outcome. It is unclear to what extent seizures during pregnancy affect subsequent psychomotor development. Older studies have shown either a negative effect on IQ or no effect [78–80]. A recent retrospective study has reported that five or more tonic-clonic seizures is a risk factor for impaired verbal IQ [50,81].

The effect of gestational exposure to anti-epileptic drugs on cognitive development

In rodents, gestational exposure to phenytoin, phenobarbitone or valproate, at doses below that needed to cause malformations, has harmful effects on behaviour and cognition [82,83]. Learning deficits, motor deficits and hyperexcitability have been observed, and there is some evidence for a critical period. In utero phenytoin exposure in monkeys appears to be more harmful for development than maternal focal seizures [84]. One study suggested carbamazepine did not have significant effects [85]. It is difficult to extrapolate these findings to humans. A recent Cochrane review emphasized the difficulty interpreting the human evidence [86]. Many studies have small sample sizes, neuropsychological methods and age at testing vary, and control of confounding factors is imperfect. A pattern does emerge despite the methodological problems. Polytherapy is more harmful than monotherapy [86].

Children of mothers with epilepsy who do not have tonic-clonic seizures and who do not take AEDs seem to have normal cognitive development [51]. Children exposed to phenytoin or carbamazepine do not seem to be developmentally different to unexposed controls at 1 year of age [87–89]. In three studies, children exposed to carbamazepine had no difference in IQ compared with controls when tested later in childhood [90–92]. One study did reveal delayed development with carbamazepine exposure compared to control, but only in some infants [93]. A number of studies have suggested that children exposed to phenytoin may have lower scores in some cognitive domains when tested later in childhood [47,91,92,94]. Another cohort, of whom 80% took phenytoin, found no such effect [79]. One study demonstrated a significantly lower IQ in children exposed to phenytoin compared with carbamazepine [95]. Most studies of exposure to phenobarbitone have not found an effect on IQ [88,96]. However, men born of mothers without epilepsy exposed to phenobarbitone in the third trimester (for various reasons) have been found to have a mean 7 points lower verbal IQ than unexposed controls [97].

Studies involving exposure to valproate cause the most concern. The evidence emerged as case series of the 'fetal valproate syndrome'. This typically included facial dysmorphism, developmental delay (especially language) and autistic behavioural phenotype [44,46]. One study found 7 of 23 (30%) valproate-exposed children had developmental delay compared with 10% of non-exposed sibs [98]. Another study reported 5 of 56 (9%) valproate-exposed infants had autistic spectrum disorder compared with 2 of 80 (2.5%) exposed to carbamazepine [99]. Children exposed to valproate in utero have also been found to have a higher incidence of additional educational needs relative to those exposed to carbamazepine or no drug [100]. Mean verbal IQ in this study was significantly lower (7 points) following gestational exposure to valproate (more than 800 mg) than carbamazepine or phenytoin or no drug [50,81]. Another study has found that adverse developmental outcomes only occurred with maternal doses of valproate above 1000 mg [64]. Similar findings have now been reported from Finland [101]. It is unclear whether, like malformations, only some infants are at risk of adverse effects on cognition. A prospective study examining differences in cognitive outcomes between AEDs is now underway (www.neadstudy.org). For the time being, we draw the conclusion that valproate poses the greatest neurodevelopmental risk, that phenytoin may present some risk and it seems least with carbamazepine. Nothing is known about the neurodevelopmental effects of the newer AEDs.

Fetal loss and growth retardation

Studies comparing stillbirth rates found higher rates in infants of mothers with epilepsy (1.3–14.0%) than in infants of mothers without epilepsy (1.1–7.8%) [102]. Fetal loss prior to 20 weeks of gestation also appears to occur more commonly in infants of mothers with epilepsy [102]. Studies show that infants born to mothers with epilepsy tend to have reduced birth weight, length and head circumference [103–105]. Reduced head circumference is especially associated with phenytoin, phenobarbitone and polytherapy and in some studies, carbamazepine [103,106]. Differences in head circumference have been noted to decrease with follow-up, and in the majority of infants these are not to be associated with long-term cognitive impairment [106,107].

The effect of pregnancy on seizure control

A recent study has provided less biased information than older case series [108]. In this report, 58% of women remained seizure free during pregnancy. About a fifth experienced an increase in seizures. Seizures were more common in those with focal epilepsy. Use of lamotrigine or oxcarbazepine was more commonly associated with deterioration in seizure control than other drugs. Tonic-clonic status epilepticus occurred in about 0.5% of pregnancies, sometimes in women who had been seizure free until then. The morbidity of status seemed less (one stillbirth and no maternal mortality) than cited in older reports [102]. Nevertheless, status epilepticus remains one of the commoner causes of maternal mortality and requires vigorous management [81]. Obstetric outcome in women with epilepsy is not different from that in the general population other than an increase in induction of labour [109].

Anti-epileptic drug pharmacokinetics during pregnancy

Decreased plasma protein binding and increased metabolism are the most important pharmacokinetic changes in pregnancy [110]. Highly protein bound drugs, like phenytoin, can undergo marked changes in total drug concentration. Studies show a reduction in total phenytoin level, starting in the first trimester and dropping by 60% in the third trimester [111,112]. Free phenytoin levels drop by 16–35% [111,112]. Some women need an increase in phenytoin dosage due to seizure exacerbation [111]. Measuring total concentrations can be misleading and free phenytoin levels should be requested if contemplating changing dosages, with a target range of 1–2 mg/L [113,114]. Total carbamazepine decreases by 10–40% in the third trimester, and free levels and carbamazepine epoxide levels do not change significantly [112,115]. Phenobarbitone (total and free) levels fall by 50% in pregnancy [112]. Total valproate levels do not change, but free levels may rise by 25% [112].

Lamotrigine levels undergo clinically important changes during pregnancy. Lamotrigine clearance (with monotherapy) increases from the first trimester and reaches more than 300% of baseline by the third trimester. Clearance may start to decrease at 32 weeks and return to baseline within 2 weeks after delivery [116,117]. Falling serum levels have been associated with an increase in seizures [108,116,118,119]. When lamotrigine was used as polytherapy with enzyme inducers, an increase in clearance of 65% was found [117]. Unfortunately the changes for an individual woman are not predictable [116,119]. Drug levels should be taken before, during and after pregnancy. Dosages may need to be increased two- to threefold during the pregnancy and restored to normal immediately after delivery. Levetiracetam clearance is slightly increased due to increased renal blood flow [120]. For other drugs that are renally excreted (gabapentin, pregabalin and vigabatrin), a similar minor increase in elimination might be predicted. Benzodiazepines in the peripartum period may produce pronounced sedative or withdrawal effects in the newborn [69,70,121]. Intravenous, but not oral, use of lorazepam near term is linked to respiratory depression, requiring ventilation in the infant [122].

Breastfeeding and anti-epileptic drugs

The use of AEDs whilst breastfeeding has recently been reviewed [113,123]. The physiological effects of AED exposure in breast milk on the infant are a function of the dose received and the infant's metabolism. The dose received is determined by mother's serum level, the protein and lipid binding of the drug and the amount of milk ingested. Phenytoin, carbamazepine, valproate and vigabatrin are not found in high concentration in breast milk (less than 50% of serum) [113]. However, idiosyncratic thrombocytopenia due to valproate in breast milk has been noted [123]. Lamotrigine, levetiracetam, ethosuximide, topiramate, phenobarbitone, gabapentin and zonisamide pass extensively into breast milk [113,124]. In the neonatal period, infant metabolism, especially glucuronidation, is under-developed and this can lead to drug accumulation. There is evidence that clinically relevant serum lamotrigine concentrations, but not adverse effects, are found in breastfed infants of mothers taking lamotrigine [125]. There appears to be active placental transport of gabapentin to the fetus, but the plasma concentration in the suckling infant is very low [126]. Serum topiramate and levetiracetam concentrations are also very low in breastfed infants, despite extensive transfer to the milk [127,128]. A mother's use of phenobarbitone or primidone has repeatedly been associated with adverse effects and should be used with care [123]. Ethosuximide concentrations in suckling infants are in the therapeutic range and side effects have been reported [123]. The transfer of benzodiazepines to breast milk is relatively low, but account has to be taken of long half-lives and caution is advised if the mother is on repeated doses [123]. Thus, most mothers can breastfeed with careful observation of the baby's well-being. Special caution is applicable if the mother takes barbiturates, benzodiazepines or ethosuximide.

The treatment of pregnant women with epilepsy

Changing treatment before conception

Preconception counselling should include confirmation of the diagnosis of epilepsy and the specific syndrome, as well as a review of treatment. A detailed account of drug choice in epilepsy is beyond the scope of this chapter [129]. Women should be offered expert advice about the teratogenicity of AED regimes and the risks to themselves, and their fetus, of seizures. Tonic-clonic seizures are potentially harmful to both mother (sudden death or accident) and infant (miscarriage and possibly developmental effects). Partial seizures may harm the mother, though there is little evidence that they are associated with adverse outcomes for the infant (excluding accidents to the mother). Simple partial seizures (auras), absences and myoclonus are very unlikely to harm mother or infant. However, because seizures preclude driving and may have occupational or social implications, women may choose to continue therapy to avoid these problems. Women who have been seizure free for one or more years should be given advice by a neurologist of syndrome-specific risk of seizure relapse on treatment withdrawal. The main risk factors are the presence of tonic-clonic and myoclonic seizures and initial difficulty controlling the epilepsy [130]. Even in low-risk cases there is a 20–30% risk of relapse within 2 years after drug withdrawal, though control is usually regained on restoring treatment [130,131]. With this information, a woman can make an informed choice whether to withdraw treatment.

Women on polytherapy need to be assessed to judge whether this is justified during pregnancy. In some circumstances, mild partial seizures, absences or myoclonus may be acceptable to allow reduction to monotherapy before conception. Women on valproate with focal epilepsy should be reassessed to judge whether conversion to a safer AED is appropriate. In generalised epilepsy, decision making is more difficult as valproate appears to offer the best seizure control [132]. Reducing the valproate dose below 1000 mg offers some reduction of teratogenic risk. A switch to lamotrigine could be considered for those who experience only tonic-clonic seizures. Myoclonus and absences may relapse on switching if these were controlled by valproate. There are insufficient data to predict what will happen to tonic-clonic seizures in the context of juvenile myoclonic epilepsy. Clearly, women must not conceive during a switch. All of these decisions require expert advice and careful discussion with the woman. All women who are planning a pregnancy should be started on 5 mg folic acid before conception. This might also be advisable for sexually active women not using contraception, or for those using less reliable methods.

During pregnancy

In general, changing treatment during pregnancy to reduce the risk of MM is misguided as most have occurred by 8 weeks of pregnancy [133]. Unfortunately, because it is not known when functional neurodevelopmental effects occur, this aspect of harm reduction remains difficult. In certain cases, with expert assessment, the dose of valproate can be lowered, or given in smaller doses more frequently, if the woman is seizure free and is still in the first trimester. It is hazardous to withdraw treatment in a woman with active epilepsy due to the risk of tonic-clonic seizures. It is not known what the best policy is for a woman seizure free on polytherapy regimes. Folic acid 5 mg daily, for at least the first trimester, should be started if not initiated preconception.

Most women do not experience a major worsening of epilepsy in pregnancy. The exception is women using AEDs whose levels change markedly in pregnancy, particularly lamotrigine. For these women, it may be helpful to know the preconception serum level associated with good seizure control, so that adjustments can be made prospectively from the first trimester. It must be remembered that for phenytoin, the total serum level falls, but the 'free level' falls less. Prospective adjustments should only be made on free levels, otherwise toxicity is a risk. Clearly, if seizure control is lost, adjustments are made on clinical grounds. A woman should be kept under review during pregnancy by the neurological team. She should be booked with an obstetric team, knowledgeable in the management of pregnancy in women with epilepsy. A high definition ultrasound should be performed around 20 weeks for malformation detection to allow for the option of therapeutic termination. The infants of women taking enzyme-inducing AEDs have an increased risk of neonatal haemorrhage (e.g., intracerebral) due to deficient clotting factors, and this can be averted with maternal oral vitamin K supplementation [134–136]. Guidelines suggest that despite the low incidence of this complication, all mothers on enzyme-inducing AEDs (carbamazepine, oxcarbazepine, phenytoin, phenobarbitone, primidone and topiramate) should be treated with 10–20 mg of vitamin K for 4 weeks before delivery [4,137]. All infants should also receive 1 mg vitamin K at birth [138].

Delivery and the puerperium

Women should present at the hospital early in labour and the paediatrician should be present at delivery if the mother has been prescribed benzodiazepines in the 4 weeks prior to delivery. Tonic-clonic seizures occur in about 1–2% of susceptible mothers. If the risk is high, oral clobazam (10–20 mg) may be given at the onset of labour. Tonic-clonic seizures should be terminated with intravenous diazepam 10 mg if they last longer than 2–3 minutes. Fetal monitoring is advisable. During labour, anti-epileptic medication is continued as normal. Neonatal AED withdrawal can present as jitteriness, seizures, apnoeic episodes, feeding difficulties and hypoglycaemia. At discharge, mothers with epilepsy should be advised on safety issues: (1) to share infant care to limit sleep deprivation (and an increased risk of seizures), (2) to sit with the baby on the floor when feeding and nappy changing, (3) never to bathe the baby alone.

Contraception

Women should be informed about AED use and contraception. Audits show that this is often poorly done [139]. Women taking enzyme-inducing AEDs (carbamazepine, oxcarbazepine, phenytoin, phenobarbitone, primidone and topiramate) need at least 50 μg ethinylestradiol in a combined oral contraceptive (COCP) to prevent pregnancy [140]. Using two pills containing 30 μg oestrogen is the most straightforward approach. A second method of contraception may be used for the first few cycles to ensure that no breakthrough bleeding occurs, which is a marker (though imperfect) of potential contraceptive failure. If this occurs, a higher dose is needed. Some guidelines suggest added protection maybe afforded by taking three packs continuously before a break, though there is no published evidence for this [4]. Despite these measures women should be advised that there is still a risk of contraceptive failure [140]. The progesterone-only pill is not recommended, though if used, double the dose should be given. The medroxyprogesterone depot injection given every 12 weeks is a suitable alternative [140]. Implants are not recommended. Oestrogens reduce lamotrigine levels by 50% [141]. Therefore, relapse of seizures may occur on starting the COCP, or toxicity on COCP withdrawal. Lamotrigine does not affect oestrogen metabolism, but does reduce levels of levonorgestrel by 12% [141]. This is not thought to be clinically relevant.

Key points

- Preconception counselling should be given to all women of childbearing age with epilepsy. It should include confirmation of the epilepsy syndrome and a review of treatment. If the diagnosis is in doubt or seizures are still occurring, women should be referred to an epilepsy specialist.
- All women should have an understanding of anti-epileptic drug teratogenesis. Treatment with a single drug is less of a risk than polytherapy. Sodium valproate appears to have a higher risk profile than other drugs.

(Continued)

(Continued)

- Some AEDs (in particular valproate) may alter intellectual and behavioural development, but our knowledge is still very incomplete.
- Folic acid 5 mg should be taken from preconception for the first trimester, though there is no proof of its protective effect in women with epilepsy.
- There is no clear evidence that minor seizures (absences, myoclonus and mild partial seizures) harm the developing fetus. Tonic-clonic seizures may do so and should be suppressed by additional drug treatment if necessary.
- Lamotrigine levels fall by 50% from the first trimester and worsening of seizures is well recognized. A pre-emptive increase in lamotrigine dose guided by serum levels may be appropriate. Total phenytoin levels fall by 50%, but free phenytoin levels (the active component) fall less. Increases in dose should be guided by free levels or clinical need. Other drugs generally do not undergo clinically relevant changes.
- Breastfeeding is generally possible with all AEDs with monitoring of the infant's well-being. Caution is appropriate with mothers on barbiturates and benzodiazepines.

References

1 Fairgrieve SD, Jackson M, Jonas P, et al. Population based, prospective study of the care of women with epilepsy in pregnancy. *BMJ* 2000;**321**:674–5.
2 Williams J, Myson V, Steward S, et al. Self-discontinuation of antiepileptic medication in pregnancy: detection by hair analysis. *Epilepsia* 2002;**43**:824–31.
3 Antiepileptics, pregnancy and the child. *Drug Ther Bull* 2005;**43**:13–16.
4 Crawford P. Best practice guidelines for the management of women with epilepsy. *Epilepsia* 2005;**46**(Suppl 9):117–24.
5 Perucca E. Birth defects after prenatal exposure to antiepileptic drugs. *Lancet Neurol* 2005;**4**:781–6.
6 Hunt SJ, Morrow JI. Safety of antiepileptic drugs during pregnancy. *Expert Opin Drug Saf* 2005;**4**:869–77.
7 Rubin P. Fortnightly review: drug treatment during pregnancy. *BMJ* 1998;**317**:1503–6.
8 Chan WY, Lorke DE, Tiu SC, et al. Proliferation and apoptosis in the developing human neocortex. *Anat Rec* 2002;**267**:261–76.
9 Caviness VS, Takahashi T, Nowakowski RS. Morphogenesis of the human cerebral cortex. In: Barth PG (ed.), *Disorders of Neuronal Migration*. London: Mac Keith press; 2003:1–23.

10 de Graaf-Peters VB, Hadders-Algra M. Ontogeny of the human central nervous system: what is happening when? *Early Hum Dev* 2006;**82**:257–66.

11 Costa LG, Steardo L, Cuomo V. Structural effects and neurofunctional sequelae of developmental exposure to psychotherapeutic drugs: experimental and clinical aspects. *Pharmacol Rev* 2004;**56**: 103–47.

12 Barrett C, Richens A. Epilepsy and pregnancy: report of an Epilepsy Research Foundation Workshop. *Epilepsy Res* 2003;**52**:147–87.

13 Danielsson BR, Skold AC, Azarbayjani F. Class III antiarrhythmics and phenytoin: teratogenicity due to embryonic cardiac dysrhythmia and reoxygenation damage. *Curr Pharm Des* 2001;**9**:787–802.

14 Dean J, Robertson Z, Yousaf S, et al. Epilepsy, fetal anticonvulsant syndrome, and polymorphisms in MTHFR and SHMT, two folate pathway genes. *Am J Hum Genet* 2003;**73**:211. (Abstract)

15 Strickler SM, Dansky LV, Miller MA, et al. Genetic predisposition to phenytoin-induced birth defects. *Lancet* 1985;**2**:746–9.

16 Faiella A, Wernig M, Consalez GG, et al. A mouse model for valproate teratogenicity: parental effects, homeotic transformations, and altered HOX expression. *Hum Mol Genet* 2000;**9**:227–36.

17 Lampen A, Carlberg C, Nau H. Peroxisome proliferator-activated receptor delta is a specific sensor for teratogenic valproic acid derivatives. *Eur J Pharmacol* 2001;**431**:25–33.

18 Finnell RH, Dansky LV. Parental epilepsy, anticonvulsant drugs, and reproductive outcome: epidemiologic and experimental findings spanning three decades; 1: animal studies. *Reprod Toxicol* 1991;**5**: 281–99.

19 Duncan S, Mercho S, Lopes-Cendes I, et al. Repeated neural tube defects and valproate monotherapy suggest a pharmacogenetic abnormality. *Epilepsia* 2001;**42**:750–3.

20 Yerby MS, Collins SD. Teratogenicity of antiepileptic drugs. In: Engel J, Pedley TA (eds.), *Epilepsy: A Comprehensive Textbook*. Philadelphia: Lippincott-Raven Publishers, 1997:1195–203.

21 Davidson DL. Discordant twins for neural tube defect on treatment with sodium valproate. *Seizure* 2002;**11**:445.

22 MRC. Prevention of neural tube defects: results of the Medical Research Council Vitamin Study. *Lancet* 1991;**338**:131–7.

23 Berry RJ, Li Z, Erickson JD, et al. Prevention of neural-tube defects with folic acid in China. *N Engl J Med* 1999;**341**:1485–90.

24 Czeizel AE, Dudas I. Prevention of the 1st occurrence of neural-tube defects by periconceptional vitamin supplementation. *N Engl J Med* 1992;**327**:1832–5.

25 Ogawa Y, Kaneko S, Otani K, et al. Serum folic acid levels in epileptic mothers and their relationship to congenital malformations. *Epilepsy Res* 1991;**8**:75–8.

26 Dansky LV, Andermann E, Rosenblatt D, et al. Anticonvulsants, folate levels, and pregnancy outcome: a prospective study. *Ann Neurol* 1987;**21**:176–82.
27 Hiilesmaa VK, Teramo K, Granstrom ML, et al. Serum folate concentrations during pregnancy in women with epilepsy: relation to antiepileptic drug concentrations, number of seizures, and fetal outcome. *Br Med J (Clin Res Ed)* 1983;**287**:577–9.
28 Hernandez-Diaz S, Werler MM, Walker AM, et al. Neural tube defects in relation to use of folic acid antagonists during pregnancy. *Am J Epidemiol* 2001;**153**:961–8.
29 Hernandez-Diaz S, Werler MM, Walker AM, et al. Folic acid antagonists during pregnancy and the risk of birth defects. *N Engl J Med* 2000;**343**:1608–14.
30 Kaaja E, Kaaja R, Hiilesmaa V. Major malformations in offspring of women with epilepsy. *Neurology* 2003;**60**:575–9.
31 Dean JC, Moore SJ, Osborne A, et al. Fetal anticonvulsant syndrome and mutation in the maternal MTHFR gene. *Clin Genet* 1999;**56**:216–20.
32 Hansen DK, Grafton TF. Lack of attenuation of valproic acid-induced effects by folinic acid in rats embryos in vitro. *Teratology* 1991;**43**:575–82.
33 Hansen DK, Grafton TF, Dial SL, et al. Effect of supplemental folic acid on valproic acid-induced embryotoxicity and tissue zinc levels in vivo. *Teratology* 1995;**52**:277–85.
34 Trotz M, Wegner C, Nau H. Valproic acid-induced neural tube defects: reduction by folinic acid in the mouse. *Life Sci* 1987;**41**:103–10.
35 Craig J, Morrison P, Morrow J, et al. Failure of periconceptual folic acid to prevent a neural tube defect in the offspring of a mother taking sodium valproate. *Seizure* 1999;**8**:253–4.
36 Wyszynski DF, Nambisan M, Surve T, et al. Increased rate of major malformations in offspring exposed to valproate during pregnancy. *Neurology* 2005;**64**:961–5.
37 Mattson RH, Gallager BB, Reynolds EH. Folate therapy in epilepsy. *Arch Neurol* 1973;**29**:78–81.
38 Dansky LV, Finnell RH. Parental epilepsy, anticonvulsant drugs, and reproductive outcome: epidemiologic and experimental findings spanning three decades; 2: human studies. *Reprod Toxicol* 1991;**5**: 301–35.
39 Lindhout D, Omtzigt JG, Cornel MC. Spectrum of neural-tube defects in 34 infants prenatally exposed to antiepileptic drugs. *Neurology* 1992;**42**:111–8.
40 Samren EB, van Duijn CM, Koch S, et al. Maternal use of antiepileptic drugs and the risk of major congenital malformations: a joint European prospective study of human teratogenesis associated with maternal epilepsy. *Epilepsia* 1997;**38**:981–90.

41 Samren EB, van Duijn CM, Christiaens GC, et al. Antiepileptic drug regimens and major congenital abnormalities in the offspring. *Ann Neurol* 1999;**46**:739–46.
42 Arpino C, Brescianini S, Robert E, et al. Teratogenic effects of antiepileptic drugs: use of an International Database on Malformations and Drug Exposure (MADRE). *Epilepsia* 2000;**41**:1436–43.
43 Rosa FW. Spina bifida in infants of women treated with carbamazepine during pregnancy. *N Engl J Med* 1991;**324**:674–7.
44 Moore SJ, Turnpenny P, Quinn A, et al. A clinical study of 57 children with fetal anticonvulsant syndromes. *J Med Genet* 2000;**37**:489–97.
45 Dean JC, Moore SJ, Turnpenny PD. Developing diagnostic criteria for the fetal anticonvulsant syndromes. *Seizure* 2000;**9**:233–4.
46 Kozma C. Valproic acid embryopathy: report of two siblings with further expansion of the phenotypic abnormalities and a review of the literature. *Am J Med Genet* 2001;**98**:168–75.
47 Hanson JW, Smith DW. The fetal hydantoin syndrome. *J Pediatr* 1975;**87**:285–90.
48 Kini U, Adab N, Vinten J, et al. Dysmorphic features: an important clue to the diagnosis and severity of fetal anticonvulsant syndromes. *Arch Dis Child Fetal Neonatal Ed* 2006;**91**:F90–5.
49 Holmes LB, Coull BA, Dorfman J, et al. The correlation of deficits in IQ with midface and digit hypoplasia in children exposed in utero to anticonvulsant drugs. *J Pediatr* 2005;**146**:118–22.
50 Vinten J, Adab N, Kini U, et al. Neuropsychological effects of exposure to anticonvulsant medication in utero. *Neurology* 2005;**64**:949–54.
51 Holmes LB, Rosenberger PB, Harvey EA, et al. Intelligence and physical features of children of women with epilepsy. *Teratology* 2000;**61**:196–202.
52 Yerby MS. Problems and management of the pregnant woman with epilepsy. *Epilepsia* 1987;**28**(Suppl 3):S29–36.
53 Canger R, Battino D, Canevini MP, et al. Malformations in offspring of women with epilepsy: a prospective study. *Epilepsia* 1999;**40**:1231–6.
54 Kaneko S, Battino D, Andermann E, et al. Congenital malformations due to antiepileptic drugs. *Epilepsy Res* 1999;**33**:145–58.
55 Holmes LB, Harvey EA, Coull BA, et al. The teratogenicity of anticonvulsant drugs. *N Engl J Med* 2001;**344**:1132–8.
56 Wide K, Winbladh B, Kallen B. Major malformations in infants exposed to antiepileptic drugs in utero, with emphasis on carbamazepine and valproic acid: a nation-wide, population-based register study. *Acta Paediatr* 2004;**93**:174–6.
57 Cunnington M, Tennis P. Lamotrigine and the risk of malformations in pregnancy. *Neurology* 2005;**64**:955–60.

58 Artama M, Auvinen A, Raudaskoski T, et al. Antiepileptic drug use of women with epilepsy and congenital malformations in offspring. *Neurology* 2005;**64**:1874–8.
59 Morrow JI, Russell A, Guthrie E, et al. Malformation risks of antiepileptic drugs in pregnancy: a prospective study from the UK Epilepsy and Pregnancy Register. *J Neurol Neurosurg Psychiatry* 2006;**77**:193–8.
60 Holmes LB, Wyszynski DF, Baldwin EJ, et al. Increased risk for non-syndromic cleft palate among infants exposed to lamotrigine during pregnancy [abstract]. *Birth Defects Res A Clin Mol Teratol* 2006;**76**:318.
61 Matalon S, Schechtman S, Goldzweig G, et al. The teratogenic effect of carbamazepine: a meta-analysis of 1255 exposures. *Reprod Toxicol* 2002;**16**:9–17.
62 Fried S, Kozer E, Nulman I, et al. Malformation rates in children of women with untreated epilepsy: a meta-analysis. *Drug Saf* 2004;**27**:197–202.
63 Alsdorf R, Wyszynski DF. Teratogenicity of sodium valproate. *Expert Opin Drug Saf* 2005;**4**:345–53.
64 Mawer G, Clayton-Smith J, Coyle H, et al. Outcome of pregnancy in women attending an outpatient epilepsy clinic: adverse features associated with higher doses of sodium valproate. *Seizure* 2002;**11**: 512–8.
65 Vajda FJ, O'Brien TJ, Hitchcock A, et al. Critical relationship between sodium valproate dose and human teratogenicity: results of the Australian register of anti-epileptic drugs in pregnancy. *J Clin Neurosci* 2004;**11**:854–8.
66 Holmes LB, Wyszynski DF, Lieberman E. The AED (antiepileptic drug) pregnancy registry: a 6-year experience. *Arch Neurol* 2004;**61**:673–8.
67 Dolovich LR, Addis A, Vaillancourt JM, et al. Benzodiazepine use in pregnancy and major malformations or oral cleft: meta-analysis of cohort and case-control studies. *BMJ* 1998;**317**:839–43.
68 Czeizel AE, Eros E, Rockenbauer M, et al. Short-term oral diazepam treatment during pregnancy – a population-based teratological case-control study. *Clin Drug Invest* 2003;**23**:451–62.
69 Iqbal MM, Sobhan T, Ryals T. Effects of commonly used benzodiazepines on the fetus, the neonate and the nursing infant. *Psychiatr Serv* 2002;**53**:39–49.
70 McElhatton PR. The effects of benzodiazepine use during pregnancy and lactation. *Reprod Toxicol* 1994;**8**:461–75.
71 Sanders DD, Stephens TD. Review of drug-induced limb defects in mammals. *Teratology* 1991;**44**:335–54.
72 Meischenguiser R, D'Giano CH, Ferraro SM. Oxcarbazepine in pregnancy: clinical experience in Argentina. *Epilepsy Behav* 2004;**5**:163–7.
73 Sahoo S, Klein P. Maternal complex partial seizure associated with fetal distress. *Arch Neurol* 2005;**62**:1304–5.

74 Paul RH, Koh KS, Bernstein SG. Changes in fetal heart rate-uterine contraction patterns associated with eclampsia. *Am J Obstet Gynecol* 1978;**130**:165–9.
75 Hiilesmaa VK, Bardy A, Teramo K. Obstetric outcome in women with epilepsy. *Am J Obstet Gynecol* 1985;**152**:499–504.
76 Teramo K, Hiilesmaa V, Bardy A, et al. Fetal heart rate during a maternal grand mal epileptic seizure. *J Perinat Med* 1979;**7**:3–6.
77 Nei M, Daly S, Liporace J. A maternal complex partial seizure in labor can affect fetal heart rate. *Neurology* 1998;**51**:904–6.
78 Majewski F, Steger M, Richter B, et al. The teratogenicity of hydantoins and barbiturates in humans, with considerations on the etiology of malformations and cerebral disturbances in the children of epileptic parents. *Int J Biol Res Pregnancy* 1981;**2**:37–45.
79 Gaily E, Kantola-Sorsa E, Granstrom ML. Intelligence of children of epileptic mothers. *J Pediatr* 1988;**113**:677–84.
80 Gaily E, Kantola-Sorsa E, Granstrom ML. Specific cognitive dysfunction in children with epileptic mothers. *Dev Med Child Neurol* 1990;**32**:403–14.
81 Adab N, Kini U, Vinten J, et al. The longer term outcome of children born to mothers with epilepsy. *J Neurol Neurosurg Psychiatry* 2004;**75**:1575–83.
82 Vorhees CV, Minck DR, Berry HK. Anticonvulsants and brain development. *Prog Brain Res* 1988;**73**:229–44
83 Hansen DK, Holson R. Developmental neurotoxicity of antiepileptic drugs. In: Slikker W, Chang LW (eds.), *Handbook of Developmental Neurotoxicology*. San Diego, CA: Academic Press; 1998:643–60.
84 Phillips NK, Lockard JS. A gestational monkey model: effects of phenytoin versus seizures on neonatal outcome. *Epilepsia* 1985;**26**: 697–703.
85 Rayburn WF, Gonzalez CL, Parker KM, et al. Chronic prenatal exposure to carbamazepine and behavior effects on mice offspring. *Am J Obstet Gynecol* 2004;**190**:517–21.
86 Adab N, Tudur SC, Vinten J, et al. Common antiepileptic drugs in pregnancy in women with epilepsy. The Cochrane Database of Systematic Reviews 2004: Art No CD004848.
87 Leavitt AM, Yerby MS, Robinson N, et al. Epilepsy in pregnancy: developmental outcome of offspring at 12 months. *Neurology* 1992;**42**: 141–3.
88 Shapiro S, Hartz SC, Siskind V, et al. Anticonvulsants and parental epilepsy in the development of birth defects. *Lancet* 1976;**1**: 272–5.
89 Wide K, Winbladh B, Tomson T, et al. Psychomotor development and minor anomalies in children exposed to antiepileptic drugs in utero: a prospective population-based study. *Dev Med Child Neurol* 2000;**42**:87–92.

90 Gaily E, Kantola-Sorsa E, Hiilesmaa V, et al. Normal intelligence in children with prenatal exposure to carbamazepine. *Neurology* 2004;**62**:28–32.

91 Rovet J, Cole S, Nulman I, et al. Effects of maternal epilepsy on children's neurodevelopment. *Child Neuropsychol* 1995;**1**:150–7.

92 Wide K, Henning E, Tomson T, et al. Psychomotor development in preschool children exposed to antiepileptic drugs in utero. *Acta Paediatr* 2002;**91**:409–14.

93 Ornoy A, Cohen E. Outcome of children born to epileptic mothers treated with carbamazepine during pregnancy. *Arch Dis Child* 1996;**75**:517–20.

94 Vanoverloop D, Schnell RR, Harvey EA, et al. The effects of prenatal exposure to phenytoin and other anticonvulsants on intellectual function at 4 to 8 years of age. *Neurotoxicol Teratol* 1992;**14**:329–35.

95 Scolnik D, Nulman I, Rovet J, et al. Neurodevelopment of children exposed in utero to phenytoin and carbamazepine monotherapy. *JAMA* 1994;**271**:767–70.

96 Hill RM, Verniaud WM, Horning MG, et al. Infants exposed in utero to antiepileptic drugs. A prospective study. *Am J Dis Child* 1974;**127**:645–53.

97 Reinisch JM, Sanders SA, Mortensen EL, et al. In utero exposure to phenobarbital and intelligence deficits in adult men. *JAMA* 1995;**274**:1518–25.

98 Dean JC, Hailey H, Moore SJ, et al. Long term health and neurodevelopment in children exposed to antiepileptic drugs before birth. *J Med Genet* 2002;**39**:251–9.

99 Rasalam AD, Hailey H, Williams JH, et al. Characteristics of fetal anticonvulsant syndrome associated autistic disorder. *Dev Med Child Neurol* 2005;**47**:551–5.

100 Adab N, Jacoby A, Smith D, et al. Additional educational needs in children born to mothers with epilepsy. *J Neurol Neurosurg Psychiatry* 2001;**70**:15–21.

101 Eriksson K, Viinikainen K, Monkkonen A, et al. Children exposed to valproate in utero – population based evaluation of risks and confounding factors for long-term neurocognitive development. *Epilepsy Res* 2005;**65**:189–200.

102 Yerby MS, Kaplan P, Tran T. Risks and management of pregnancy in women with epilepsy. *Cleve Clin J Med* 2004;**71**(Suppl 2):S25–37.

103 Wide K, Winbladh B, Tomson T, et al. Body dimensions of infants exposed to antiepileptic drugs in utero: observations spanning 25 years. *Epilepsia* 2000;**41**:854–61.

104 Hvas CL, Henriksen TB, Ostergaard JR, et al. Epilepsy and pregnancy: effect of antiepileptic drugs and lifestyle on birthweight. *BJOG* 2000;**107**:896–902.

105 Battino D, Kaneko S, Andermann E, et al. Intrauterine growth in the offspring of epileptic women: a prospective multicenter study. *Epilepsy Res* 1999;**36**:53–60.

106 Dessens AB, Cohen-Kettenis PT, Mellenbergh GJ, et al. Association of prenatal phenobarbital and phenytoin exposure with small head size at birth and with learning problems. *Acta Paediatr* 2000;**89**:533–41.

107 Hirano T, Fujioka T, Okada J, et al. Physical and psychomotor development in the offspring born to mothers with epilepsy. *Epilepsia* 2004;**45**:53–7.

108 The EURAP Study Group. Seizure control and treatment in pregnancy. Observations from the EURAP epilepsy pregnancy registry. *Neurology* 2006;**66**:354–60.

109 Richmond JR, Krishnamoorthy P, Andermann E, et al. Epilepsy and pregnancy: an obstetric perspective. *Am J Obstet Gynecol* 2004;**190**:371–9.

110 Pennell PB. Antiepileptic drug pharmacokinetics during pregnancy and lactation. *Neurology* 2003;**61**:S35–42.

111 Tomson T, Lindbom U, Ekqvist B, et al. Epilepsy and pregnancy: a prospective study of seizure control in relation to free and total plasma concentrations of carbamazepine and phenytoin. *Epilepsia* 1994;**35**:122–30.

112 Yerby MS, Friel PN, McCormick K. Antiepileptic drug disposition during pregnancy. *Neurology* 1992;**42**:12–6.

113 Tomson T. Gender aspects of pharmacokinetics of new and old AEDs – pregnancy and breast-feeding. *Ther Drug Monit* 2005;**27**:718–21.

114 Burt M, Anderson DC, Kloss J, et al. Evidence-based implementation of free phenytoin therapeutic drug monitoring. *Clin Chem* 2000;**46**:1132–5.

115 Tomson T, Lindbom U, Ekqvist B, et al. Disposition of carbamazepine and phenytoin in pregnancy. *Epilepsia* 1994;**35**:131–5.

116 Pennell PB, Newport DJ, Stowe ZN, et al. The impact of pregnancy and childbirth on the metabolism of lamotrigine. *Neurology* 2004;**62**:292–5.

117 Tran TA, Leppik IE, Blesi K, et al. Lamotrigine clearance during pregnancy. *Neurology* 2002;**59**:251–5.

118 de Haan GJ, Edelbroek P, Segers J, et al. Gestation-induced changes in lamotrigine pharmacokinetics: a monotherapy study. *Neurology* 2004;**63**:571–3.

119 Petrenaite V, Sabers A, Hansen-Schwartz J. Individual changes in lamotrigine plasma concentrations during pregnancy. *Epilepsy Res* 2005;**65**:185–8.

120 Pennell PB, Kognati A, Helmers SL, et al. The impact of pregnancy and childbirth on the elimination of levetiracetam. *Epilepsia* 2005;**46**:89–9.

121 Swortfiguer D, Cissoko H, Giraudeau B, et al. Neonatal consequences of benzodiazepines used during the last month of pregnancy. *Arch Pediatr* 2005;**12**:1327–31.

122 Whitelaw AGL, Cummings AJ, McFadyen IR. Effect of maternal lorazepam on the neonate. *BMJ* 1981;**282**:1106–8.
123 Hagg S, Spigset O. Anticonvulsant use during lactation. *Drug Saf* 2000;**22**:425–40.
124 Kawada K, Itoh S, Kusaka T, et al. Pharmacokinetics of zonisamide in perinatal period. *Brain Dev* 2002;**24**:95–7.
125 Liporace J, Kao A, D'Abreu A. Concerns regarding lamotrigine and breast-feeding. *Epilepsy Behav* 2004;**5**:102–5.
126 Ohman I, Vitols S, Tomson T. Pharmacokinetics of gabapentin during delivery, in the neonatal period, and lactation: does a fetal accumulation occur during pregnancy? *Epilepsia* 2005;**46**:1621–4.
127 Johannessen SI, Helde G, Brodtkorb E. Levetiracetam concentrations in serum and in breast milk at birth and during lactation. *Epilepsia* 2005;**46**:775–7.
128 Ohman I, Vitols S, Luef G, et al. Topiramate kinetics during delivery, lactation, and in the neonate: preliminary observations. *Epilepsia* 2002;**43**:1157–60.
129 McCorry D, Chadwick D, Marson A. Current drug treatment of epilepsy in adults. *Lancet Neurol* 2004;**3**:729–35.
130 Chadwick D, Bessant P, Eaton B, et al. Prognostic index for recurrence of seizures after remission of epilepsy. *Br Med J* 1993;**306**: 1374–8.
131 Chadwick D, Taylor J, Johnson T. Outcomes after seizure recurrence in people with well-controlled epilepsy and the factors that influence it. The MRC Antiepileptic Drug Withdrawal Group. *Epilepsia* 1996;**37**:1043–50.
132 Nicolson A, Appleton RE, Chadwick DW, et al. The relationship between treatment with valproate, lamotrigine, and topiramate and the prognosis of the idiopathic generalised epilepsies. *J Neurol Neurosurg Psychiatry* 2004;**75**:75–9.
133 Moore K, Persaud T. *Before We Are Born: Essentials of Embryology and Birth Defects*. Philadelphia: Saunders; 2003.
134 Cornelissen M, Steegers-Theunissen R, Kollee L, et al. Increased incidence of neonatal vitamin K deficiency resulting from maternal anticonvulsant therapy. *Am J Obstet Gynecol* 1993;**168**:923–8.
135 Cornelissen M, Steegers-Theunissen R, Kollee L, et al. Supplementation of vitamin K in pregnant women receiving anticonvulsant therapy prevents neonatal vitamin K deficiency. *Am J Obstet Gynecol* 1993;**168**:884–8.
136 Moslet U, Hansen ES. A review of vitamin K, epilepsy and pregnancy. *Acta Neurol Scand* 1992;**85**:39–43.
137 Practice parameter: management issues for women with epilepsy (summary statement). Report of the Quality Standards Subcommittee of the American Academy of Neurology. *Epilepsia* 1998;**39**:1226–31.

138 American Academy of Pediatrics. Controversies concerning vitamin K and the newborn. American Academy of Pediatrics Committee on Fetus and Newborn. *Pediatrics* 2003;**112**:191–2.

139 Bell GS, Nashef L, Kendall S, et al. Information recalled by women taking anti-epileptic drugs for epilepsy: a questionnaire study. *Epilepsy Res* 2002;**52**:139–46.

140 Faculty of family planning and reproductive health care. FFPRHC Guidance (April 2005). Drug interactions with hormonal contraception. *J Fam Plann Reprod Health Care* 2005;**31**:139–51.

141 Sidhu J, Job S, Singh S, et al. The pharmacokinetic and pharmacodynamic consequences of the co-administration of lamotrigine and a combined oral contraceptive in healthy female subjects. *Br J Clin Pharmacol* 2006;**61**:191–9.

CHAPTER 10

Treatment of diabetes in pregnancy

Nick Vaughan, Kate Morel, Louise Walker

Introduction

Diabetes is probably the most common disorder that influences the outcome of pregnancy. Two to three women per thousand of reproductive age are known to have type 1 diabetes before conception and a further significant proportion of pregnancies in otherwise normal women may be complicated by gestational diabetes. However, with the dramatically increasing prevalence of type 2 diabetes, more than a quarter of all pre-gestational diabetic pregnancies are occurring in this group. Type 2 diabetes is strongly associated with social deprivation and belonging to a minority ethnic group. It carries as great a risk of adverse outcome for the baby as type 1 diabetes.

In the UK, babies of women with type 1 or type 2 diabetes are almost five times more likely to be stillborn and nearly three times as likely to die in the first month of life as those of mothers without these conditions. They have double the risk of having a major congenital malformation. These statistics are from the recent Confidential Enquiry into Maternal and Child Health [1] (CEMACH report). This has highlighted the need to ensure that women with diabetes receive an effective service that integrates pre-pregnancy counselling, primary care responsibilities and essential specialist care. It underlines the importance of striving to achieve the standards set by the Diabetes National Service Framework (NSF) [2] and the NSF for Children, Young People and Maternity Services [3]. The goal for diabetes in pregnancy, as originally voiced 15 years

---

Prescribing in Pregnancy, 4th edition. Edited by Peter Rubin and Margaret Ramsay,
 ISBN: 978-1-4051-4712-5.

ago in the St Vincent Declaration [4], remains 'to achieve pregnancy outcomes in the woman with diabetes that approximates that of the non-diabetic woman'.

Pregnancy is a high-risk state for both the woman with diabetes and the fetus, and the importance of good metabolic control in pregnant women with diabetes is undisputed. The complications such as macrosomia, neonatal hypoglycaemia, miscarriage, intrauterine death and hydramnios, as well as increased perinatal mortality rate and neonatal morbidity, can be minimised by intensive efforts to achieve strict normoglycaemia. A few centres now report perinatal mortality in the babies of women with insulin-dependent diabetes approaching the rate found in the normal population, but it is disappointing that this does not seem more widely achievable. It must also not be forgotten that the usual complications of pregnancy such as infection, hydramnios, pre-eclampsia and placental insufficiency may also occur more frequently, and some specific diabetic complications, particularly retinopathy, may develop or progress rapidly during gestation. Furthermore, the increased rate of major congenital malformations compared to non-diabetic pregnancies directly relates to metabolic control in the few months before and at the time of conception.

In the organisation and delivery of diabetes care in pregnancy, great emphasis is placed upon a multidisciplinary team approach, the team comprising diabetologist, obstetrician, diabetes nurse specialist, midwife, dietitian, neonatologist and, most importantly, the patient herself. Preconception education and counselling for women with pre-gestational diabetes, the use of intensive home blood glucose monitoring to achieve optimal glycaemic control, rigorous maternal and fetal surveillance with individualised timing and mode of delivery are central to reducing adverse outcomes of pregnancy with diabetes.

It is accepted that good glycaemic control should be achieved prior to and during pregnancy in order to reduce the risk of adverse outcomes. Elevated blood glucose levels in the preconception period are associated with higher rates of miscarriage and major congenital malformations [5–7]. Glycosylated haemoglobin (HbA1c) should be used to monitor long-term glycaemic control. During the preconception period and throughout pregnancy it is recommended that the HbA1c should be within the normal non-diabetic range. One of the most important decisions therefore is the choice of insulin treatment both before and during pregnancy.

Each patient must have an insulin regimen that provides sufficient flexibility to maintain a normal blood glucose concentration throughout the day and night, without serious hypoglycaemia, and that will also accommodate increasing insulin requirements as gestation progresses. This chapter outlines the management of diabetes for women with established diabetes, both type 1 and type 2, as well as for those with gestational diabetes who require insulin therapy. It must not be forgotten that in many countries pregnant women with type 2 diabetes substantially outnumber those with type 1, and an increasing prevalence is being seen in the UK. Some patients with previously unrecognised type 2 diabetes may present during pregnancy. However, the identification of gestational diabetes is not discussed as this is not without controversy and is well discussed elsewhere [8,9].

Metabolic changes in normal and diabetic pregnancy

Essential to the management of diabetes in pregnancy is an understanding of the metabolic changes that occur in mothers without diabetes. Plasma glucose concentrations remain remarkably constant, although at slightly lower levels than in the non-pregnant state. This is despite increasing insulin resistance due to changes in the hormonal environment, including rising levels of oestrogen, progesterone and human placental lactogen. Enhanced insulin secretion is able to compensate for these changes, but where there is inadequate functional islet-cell reserve to meet these increased insulin requirements, gestational diabetes will develop. As some 50% of patients with gestational diabetes develop non-insulin-dependent diabetes later in life, it seems likely that they already have an intrinsic β-cell defect.

Initially the metabolic adaptations of pregnancy are concerned with increased energy storage, and most of the early weight gain seen in pregnancy is the consequence of fat deposition. However, the substrate demands of the fetus gradually increase and by the end of the second trimester these are substantial. As a result there is increasing loss of glucose to the fetus and accelerated maternal fat mobilisation, leading to modestly increased plasma non-esterified fatty acid and ketone levels. This is sometimes referred to as 'accelerated starvation' [10]. In the patient with diabetes, this preferential transfer of glucose to the fetus is particularly damaging to the mother's metabolic control unless there is an adequate compensatory increase in dietary carbohydrate.

The fetal β cell is not ordinarily stimulated by physiological changes of glucose, but when maternal diabetes is poorly regulated the fetus is exposed to much higher levels than usual. This increased metabolite delivery stimulates the fetal islet, causing hyperinsulinaemia and β-cell hyperplasia. Facilitated diffusion of glucose across the placenta becomes saturated at about 11 mmol/L, so that the rate of transfer of glucose to the fetus does not increase when maternal blood glucose rises beyond this level. Thus, the beneficial effects of maternal blood glucose control are only seen below about 10 mmol/L. Improvement of control from 'bad' to 'average' will have little physiological effect on glucose transport and will be of no benefit to fetal development and progress. Fetal hyperinsulinaemia directly leads to macrosomia, it may inhibit lung maturation and surfactant production, and enhanced β-cell responsiveness following delivery may result in persistent hypoglycaemia.

Organisation of diabetic care in pregnancy

Care should be focused in units specialising in management of pregnancy with diabetes and is best delivered by a multidisciplinary team comprising a diabetologist and obstetrician with a special interest in pregnancy and diabetes, a diabetes nurse specialist, dietitian, neonatologist and ophthalmologist. Patients should be seen regularly and frequently (at least fortnightly, with telephone contact in between, until 34 weeks and then weekly), before, during and after pregnancy. Joint clinics, with an obstetrician, diabetologist, diabetes nurse specialist and dietitian liaising closely, are the optimal arrangement. Those women developing gestational diabetes should receive the same level of care.

Preconception counselling

Ideally, pregnancies in women with diabetes should be planned. Discussion about the need for good glycaemic control prior to and during pregnancy should preferably take place before any attempts to conceive. The majority of women with type 2 diabetes will require insulin, and some preparation for this may be necessary before conception is contemplated. For overweight women with type

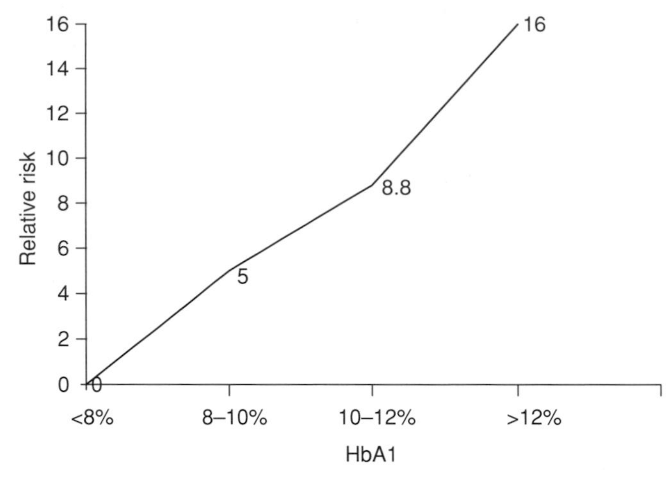

Figure 10.1 Relative risk of congenital malformation in diabetic pregnancy related to HbA1 at conception.

2 diabetes or previous gestational diabetes, it is also an opportunity for dietetic review to encourage changes to diet and lifestyle to help them to improve glycaemic control and achieve weight loss prior to conception. Both intensified glycaemic control and weight loss preconceptually can improve pregnancy outcome [11].

Congenital malformations are common in pregnancies in type 2 diabetes, but this probably just reflects the level of glycaemic control in early pregnancy. Despite the dramatic reductions of many of the complications related to poor metabolic control, the incidence of congenital malformations in children of mothers with diabetes remains two to three times greater than the incidence in the general population. Fetal anomalies and multiple malformations still occur more frequently than in the normal population. This has been shown to be directly related to HbA1 levels at the time of conception [12] (Figure 10.1). Organogenesis for all sites in which the congenital anomalies of children of mothers with diabetes are most common is essentially complete within the first 6 weeks of gestation, before the mother may realise she is even pregnant. Pregnancy should thus ideally be deferred until prolonged good metabolic control has been attained. Evidence of this would generally be taken as an HbA1c in the normal non-diabetic range. Women with diabetes have an increased risk of fetal neural tube defects and should be offered pre-pregnancy folic acid supplements (5 mg daily) [13–16], continuing up to 12 weeks of gestation.

Management of diabetes in pregnancy

Nutritional management

Adequate dietary modification is perhaps the single most important aspect of pregnancy management in the context of diabetes. Without this, achieving near-normal glycaemic control may prove to be very difficult or impossible. The aims of nutrition therapy and dietetic advice during pregnancy are, therefore:

- Optimising glycaemic control
- Ensuring adequate nutrition for mother and fetus
- Providing guidance on food safety and food avoidance specific to pregnancy
- Managing problems common to pregnancy that can influence dietary intake or nutritional requirements
- Managing weight gain.

There is consensus that all women with diabetes (type 1 or type 2) should receive preconceptual advice from a registered dietitian, and then regularly throughout the pregnancy within the specialist multidisciplinary team. This is especially important for those with pre-existing type 1 diabetes as they are very likely to self-adjust their mealtime insulin doses according to the carbohydrate content of their meals, planned physical activity and pre-meal blood glucose values. Women with gestational diabetes should also have access to advice from a dietitian. Improved pregnancy outcome has been demonstrated in the Australian Carbohydrate Intolerance Study in Pregnant Women trial in those who received individualised dietary advice from a registered dietitian as part of their management [17]. Dietetic consultations also provide the opportunity to discuss breastfeeding, weight management postpartum and, for women with gestational diabetes, diet and lifestyle advice to reduce risk of developing diabetes in the future.

To optimise glycaemic control, adequate carbohydrate distributed through regular meals and snacks (between meals and at bedtime) is recommended for all women with diabetes in pregnancy, including those with gestational diabetes. This is important to help prevent hypoglycaemic episodes, maintain insulin sensitivity and avoid 'starvation ketosis'. Inevitably, where insulin is being used to achieve strict glycaemic control, the risk of hypoglycaemia will be greater and the fear of hypoglycaemia becomes a potential barrier to reaching the required blood glucose targets. Inclusion of low glycaemic index carbohydrate foods may help to improve glycaemic control. Low glycaemic index choices can help to increase insulin sensitivity, reduce risk of hypoglycaemia and ketosis, and reduce postprandial hyperglycaemia during pregnancy [11]. If women are overweight, or have had excessive weight gain during pregnancy, they will need guidance on appropriate low-fat, carbohydrate-rich snacks, such as fruit, low-fat yoghurt and dried fruit.

The diet during pregnancy must be nutritionally adequate. This is no different for women with pre-existing diabetes or gestational diabetes. There are extra requirements for certain nutrients during pregnancy. Although some of these will be met by increased absorption and reduced losses, a dietary assessment by a dietitian, preferably preconceptually, can identify women at risk and appropriate dietary changes or supplementation can be advised. Folate supplementation up to 12 weeks of gestation is essential. In general, food choices that are rich in nutrients should be encouraged (such as fruit, vegetables, wholegrains, lean meats, low-fat dairy products) instead of foods that are high in calories, fat and sugar and those with little nutritional value (such as cakes, pastries).

The Food Standards Agency regularly reviews and updates its advice for pregnancy, and these specific recommendations are available on their website (http://www.eatwell.gov.uk). The guidance can be categorised into advice regarding food hygiene to prevent food contamination during pregnancy and that to avoid or limit foods that may contain pollutants or allergens, due to the risk of food poisoning or because of their vitamin A, caffeine or alcohol content.

Nausea, sickness, heartburn, constipation, anaemia are common problems in pregnancy. For women with diabetes, these can be particularly troublesome as they may adversely affect glycaemic control as well as nutritional intake. In many cases, advice regarding food choices and eating patterns may be sufficient to relieve these problems, at least to an extent that allows the achievement of an adequate nutritional intake. However, some women with type 1 diabetes with severe nausea or hyperemesis gravidarum may require some form of nutritional support to prevent hypoglycaemia or ketoacidosis. These women will require input from the specialist team that includes a dietitian.

Whenever possible, overweight women with known type 1 or type 2 diabetes should be encouraged to lose weight preconceptually [18], although active weight loss during pregnancy is not encouraged for risk of compromising nutrition and fetal growth. Recommendations for appropriate weight gain in pregnancy are between 7 and 16 kg [19], based on the pre-pregnancy body mass index, and it may be suggested that lower fat, nutrient-rich choices are substituted for high-fat, high-calorie options to prevent excessive weight gain during pregnancy. There is, however, a lack of consensus around the optimal energy, carbohydrate and fat composition of diets for women with gestational diabetes, although low-calorie diets are not currently recommended [18]. Overweight women who have had gestational diabetes should be encouraged to continue with healthy eating habits postpartum, to achieve weight loss, to reduce their risk of developing gestational diabetes in subsequent pregnancies and reduce the risk of type 2 diabetes in later life.

Insulin treatment

Several factors must be considered when selecting an insulin regimen. Any regimen must be able to take account of the substantial changes in insulin sensitivity that may increase daily doses of insulin severalfold as pregnancy progresses. Regular home blood glucose measurements are essential not only to meet the day-to-day variations in blood glucose concentrations but also to keep up with increasing insulin requirements. These should be undertaken with a home blood glucose meter with a memory (a useful check of compliance). With this degree of surveillance and the patient's almost invariably higher motivation, it is possible to achieve sufficiently good control with most insulin regimens that entail two or more injections of a mixture of insulins. However, the use of multiple injections ('basal bolus regimens') has become common practice. Substantial changes in strategy are best initiated pre-pregnancy.

Choice of insulin regimens

It is preferable to use human insulin in diabetic pregnancy, although a very small minority of patients who are still using animal insulins, because of hypoglycaemic unawareness, may be reluctant to change. Porcine insulin is probably acceptable but bovine insulin is best avoided as it can produce significant levels of insulin antibodies that freely cross the placenta. These have been implicated as a cause of infant morbidity, possibly affecting β-cell function of the fetus and influencing neonatal insulin secretion. Whilst the current insulin analogues possess theoretically attractive properties for pregnancy, none are licensed for use in pregnancy. Some of the short-acting analogues are being used more widely, seemingly without problems.

Once daily insulin regimens

These would seldom be appropriate in pregnant mothers with diabetes established before pregnancy, but single daily injections of an intermediate-duration insulin before breakfast may be very effective in some women with type 2 or mild gestational diabetes. Such individuals can usually produce sufficient insulin in a fasting state overnight to maintain normoglycaemia and thus an intermediate insulin, e.g., an isophane, such as Humulin I (Lilly), Insulatard (Novo-Nordisk) would be suitable. Additional short-acting or soluble insulin, e.g., Actrapid (Novo-Nordisk) or Humulin S (Lilly) may be added later as a fast-acting component to counter postprandial hyperglycaemia. The use of such regimens significantly reduces the incidence of fetal macrosomia in women with gestational diabetes when compared with treatment by diet alone [20].

The newer short-acting insulin analogues insulin lispro (Humalog (Lilly)) and insulin aspart (Novorapid (Novo-Nordisk)) have rapid absorption characteristics that provide a peak insulin concentration more rapidly than obtained with human insulin. This results in lower postprandial plasma glucose concentrations [21,22]. This is therapeutically attractive in the context of the increased insulin resistance associated with pregnancy. However, it is unknown whether these analogue insulins are teratogenic. Maternally derived insulin can only cross the placenta if antibody bound. In clinical trials with insulin lispro, there has been no observed increase in antibody response. This means little insulin transfer from mother to fetus and thus no likely increased risk for congenital malformations [21,23]. A multicentre, multinational study in 500 pregnancies exposed to insulin lispro (Humalog) during organogenesis showed no increase in malformation rates [24].

Anxieties have been expressed that the use of insulin lispro during pregnancies complicated by diabetes may accelerate retinopathy through its influence on the IGF-1 (insulin-like growth factor 1) system [25]. This seems unlikely as insulin lispro binds to the IGF-1 receptor with an affinity of only about 1/1000 that of IGF-1 and with an affinity of only about 1.5 times human insulin. Insulin aspart (Novorapid) has only 69% IGF-1 activity that of human insulin. Whilst remaining unlicensed for use in pregnancy, these analogues are being used increasingly in some centres.

Twice daily combinations of short- and intermediate-acting insulins

This type of regimen is still fairly widely used outside pregnancy – although diminishing in preference to basal prandial regimens – and is perfectly capable of providing adequate control during pregnancy as well. The usual combinations are a soluble insulin with an isophane insulin. Pre-mixed formulations of these insulins should be avoided in pregnancy as they do not afford sufficient flexibility. It is preferable to change women using these to free-mixing their insulins during the preconception period. The ability to change the proportion of short- to intermediate-acting insulin is important because as pregnancy progresses, the required balance between the two may change with increasing insulin resistance. Frequently it is found that hyperglycaemia before breakfast cannot be resolved by increasing the evening dose of isophane insulin without incurring frequent hypoglycaemia during the night, partly as a result of continued glucose usage in the fetoplacental unit. The general solution to this is to divide the evening injection, taking the short-acting insulin with the evening meal and the intermediate insulin at bedtime. Similarly, as gestation progresses, the proportion of short-acting insulin required may increase, reflecting increased insulin resistance, and to control postprandial hyperglycaemia in the afternoon it often becomes necessary to abandon the morning dose of intermediate insulin in preference to an additional lunch-time injection of short-acting insulin. From 36-week onwards, there is a tendency for the fasting blood glucose concentration to fall, which may require reduction or even omission of the evening injection of intermediate insulin. Sudden dramatic falls in insulin requirements at this time should alert the clinicians to the possibility of placental insufficiency sufficient to threaten the pregnancy.

Multiple daily insulin injections

Many younger patients with diabetes already employ such regimens, using pen-type insulin delivery devices. It is a particularly satisfactory means of achieving excellent metabolic control which is readily understood by the patient and can easily be altered to cope with variations in diet and activity. Generally, a short-acting insulin is administered with each of the main meals of the day and an isophane is given at bedtime. Close self-monitoring is essential for this type of regimen, but this will not differ from what is required for pregnancy anyway. Unfortunately, glargine insulin (Lantus (Sanofi-Aventis)), whilst commonly used in both type 1 and type 2 diabetes, is unlicensed for pregnancy and in view of theoretical considerations is not being recommended for use in pregnancy. It has a sixfold higher binding affinity for IGF-1 receptors, and experimental studies suggest an increased mitogenicity on tumour cell lines at high dosage. Until large-scale studies have demonstrated that placental transfer of glargine insulin is similar to the transfer of human insulin, and there is no increased risk to the fetus, this agent is not recommended. Its use is perhaps only justified where severe hypoglycaemia has been a problem, and there must be full discussion of the safety issues with the patient. Furthermore, this means that patients established on glargine insulin have to be switched back to an isophane basal insulin in the preconception period, or immediately an unplanned pregnancy is detected. Detimir insulin (Levemir (Novo-Nordisk)), another long-acting insulin analogue, does not have increased IGF-1 activity, so may eventually prove to be an attractive long-acting insulin alternative, but again is currently unlicensed for use in pregnancy.

Continuous subcutaneous insulin infusion

Open-loop subcutaneous insulin infusion with miniature pumps can achieve near-normal glycaemic control in appropriately selected patients. However, multiple injection regimens remain a simpler solution that can achieve very similar results and continuous subcutaneous insulin infusion is potentially more dangerous in pregnancy. Severe hypoglycaemia is a significant risk and the rapid development of ketoacidosis may occur in the event of pump failure. This option should be considered very carefully and probably only undertaken in centres with extensive pump experience.

Oral hypoglycaemic agents

Commonly, women with type 2 diabetes are taking sulphonylureas and/or metformin prior to conception. Hitherto, these have little place in the management of diabetes in pregnancy, although the use of metformin has been attracting increasing interest in recent years. The main anxiety about sulphonylureas in pregnancy is the possibility of further increasing the degree of fetal hyperinsulinaemia by direct drug-induced stimulation. Sulphonylureas, with the exception of glyburide [26], cross the placenta and have been implicated as a direct cause of neonatal hypoglycaemia [27]. The long-acting agent chlorpropamide is particularly dangerous and should not be used in the last 4 weeks of gestation. There is no convincing evidence that these drugs are teratogenic. Metformin, which does not cross the placenta, has been reported to be useful in some obese individuals with type 2 diabetics who are inadequately controlled by diet [28]. There are a range of theoretical and practical benefits from using metformin therapy instead of insulin therapy in later pregnancy, but there is insufficient data currently to support its routine usage. Several reports of the use of metformin during pregnancy in women with polycystic ovary syndrome have not shown adverse pregnancy outcomes. In these women, taking metformin before, during the first trimester or throughout pregnancy [29–32] reduced rates of spontaneous abortion and normal growth development, and normal maternal morbidity and mortality rates are observed. There is also a reduced subsequent risk of gestational diabetes with continued use of metformin during pregnancy [33]. Most authorities, however, continue to recommend that metformin is not routinely used except where any potential harm is outweighed by the benefits of metformin usage, e.g., severe insulin resistance or refusal to use insulin. Glitazones are unlicensed for use in pregnancy and are not recommended.

Targets for monitoring of metabolic control

The mean diurnal blood glucose concentration in non-diabetic pregnant women is around 5 mmol/L at 30 weeks of gestation [34]. Diabetic women should be aiming for this level of control, attempting to obtain fasting and preprandial values of between 4 and 6 mmol/L [35] and postprandial values of less than 10 mmol/L. This will be reflected in an HbA1c value within the normal non-diabetic range, certainly <7% and preferably close to 6%. It must not be forgotten that there is also a physiological reduction in glycaemic values observed by around 20 weeks of gestation. This reduction in HbA1c levels is due to the increased haematopoiesis and the presence of unglycated red cells in the circulation in pregnancy. Health professionals and women may frequently be unaware of this pattern and may falsely attribute this physiological shift to an improvement in control.

Home blood glucose measurement is an essential routine aspect of self-management and should be performed 4–6 times/day to recognise the need for insulin dose modification. This dosage adjustment can be performed by the medical team, but the patient should be encouraged and helped to gain the confidence to undertake this herself. Continuous blood glucose profiling may be a useful additional tool to assessing and optimising glycaemic control. HbA1c levels should be measured regularly as this provides an objective assessment of glycaemic control. Target values should be the middle of the normal non-diabetic range.

Hypoglycaemia is an inevitable consequence of achieving strict glycaemic control. All women on insulin should therefore be provided with glucagon 1 mg (Lilly) or GlucaGen (Novo-Nordisk) for use in moderate to severe hypoglycaemia and their relatives should be instructed in its use.

Management of labour

Dramatic changes in insulin sensitivity may occur in insulin-dependent diabetics at the time of delivery. Once active labour has started, insulin requirements fall. After delivery, once the placenta and its hormonal products have been removed, there is a further rapid reduction in insulin requirement. Indeed, immediately after delivery, insulin requirements may fall below pre-pregnancy values.

During labour the simplest scheme is to use a constant infusion of 10% glucose at a rate of 1 L every 8 hours. An independent insulin infusion of human soluble insulin, initially at 1 unit/h, is also given; this is subsequently adjusted on the basis of hourly bedside blood glucose [35]. This system may be used irrespective of the last subcutaneous insulin dose, but where induction of labour or caesarean section is planned it is best started at breakfast time after a bedtime injection of isophane insulin. As soon as the infant is delivered, the insulin infusion must be reduced or, in women with gestational diabetes, stopped altogether. The glucose infusion is continued until the next meal in patients who had vaginal deliveries or until a normal diet is resumed in those delivered by caesarean section. The pre-pregnancy insulin doses should be resumed at this time and adjusted according to the blood sugar levels. An additional 40–50 g carbohydrate, relative to the pre-pregnancy dietary intake, is generally recommended during lactation. Women should also be warned about the potential risk of hypoglycaemia whilst feeding, especially in the middle of the night. They may need advice on appropriate snacks or fluids that contain carbohydrate. Oral hypoglycaemic agents, where they were being used before pregnancy, are probably best avoided. Small quantities of sulphonylureas are secreted into breast milk and therefore can theoretically induce hypoglycaemia in the infant. This is probably of significance only with the longer acting sulphonylureas such as chlorpropamide. Metformin is not recommended for use in lactation. However, there is no evidence of harm for the infant from the small amount of metformin that is secreted into breast milk [36]. Infant exposure to metformin can be minimised by breastfeeding just before taking the dose and by avoiding feeding for at least 2–3 hours after taking the dose. It has been suggested that prophylactic antibiotics should be given after operative deliveries to offset the increased risk of wound infection in women with diabetes [35].

Treatment of diabetic ketoacidosis

Pregnant women with diabetes are much more prone to diabetic ketoacidosis due to the combination of insulin resistance and accelerated catabolism of pregnancy. Initiating factors are the same as those for any person with diabetes and include vomiting, infections, failure of insulin administration or failure to meet increasing insulin requirements. Ketoacidosis in pregnancy must be treated with the utmost urgency as fetal loss occurs in almost 50% of cases. Patients are best managed on a medical intensive care unit along conventional lines but with close fetal monitoring. Adequate fluid and potassium replacement is essential in conjunction with intravenous insulin infusion, adjusted to achieve a smooth reduction of plasma glucose concentration. Initial rehydration should be with normal saline; this should be changed to 10% dextrose, once the blood glucose is less than 10 mmol/L and continued until the patient is free of ketones.

The use of corticosteroids in premature labour before 34 weeks of gestation to accelerate fetal lung maturation may dramatically increase insulin resistance. Similarly, the use of intravenous β sympathomimetic agents to treat premature uterine contractions will cause severe hyperglycaemia and ketoacidosis unless appropriately anticipated. Careful glucose monitoring should always accompany this form of treatment and aggressive intravenous insulin treatment must be started if necessary.

Conclusions

Whilst considerable improvements in the prognosis for pregnancy complicated by diabetes have been achieved in the past two or three decades, the recent CEMACH report [1] has shown that diabetes care during pregnancy is still very variable and adverse outcomes are still well in excess of those in pregnancies not complicated by diabetes. All groups of women, regardless of type or ethnic group, should be entering pregnancy with substantially better glycaemic control. This has followed the recognition of the need for achieving near normoglycaemia, not only during pregnancy but also in the preconception period. The multidisciplinary team approach is central to success. The choice of insulin regimen may at first appear bewilderingly diverse, whether two, three or four injections a day, but it is important only in so far as it meets the patient's individual requirements to achieve normoglycaemia safely and without serious hypoglycaemia. No regimen is ideal; much depends upon the patient's co-operation and understanding. Complex regimens are not a substitute for education and careful monitoring of diabetes.

Key points

- Aim for good glycaemic control preconceptually
- Give diabetic women who are contemplating pregnancy 5 mg folic acid daily
- The aim of all insulin regimens is to achieve normoglycaemia safely, without serious hypoglycaemia
- Oral hypoglycaemic agents are not recommended for use in pregnancy

References

1 Confidential Enquiry into Maternal and Child Health. Pregnancy in women with type 1 and type 2 diabetes in 2002–03, England, Wales and Northern Ireland. London: CEMACH; 2005.

2 Diabetes National Service Framework Delivery Strategy, 2003. Available at: http://www.dh.gov.uk/PolicyAndGuidance/HealthAndSocial Care-Topics/Diabetes/fs/en.

3 National Service Framework for Children, Young people and Maternity Services, 2004. Available at: http://www.dh.gov.uk/PolicyAndGuidance/HealthAndSocialCareTopics/ChildrenServices/fs/en.

4 Krans HMJ, Porta M, Keen H (eds.). *Diabetes Care and Research in Europe: The St Vincent Declaration Action Programme*. Copenhagen: WHO; 1992.

5 Diabetes Control and Complications Trial Research Group. Pregnancy outcomes in the Diabetes Control and Complications Trial. *Am J Obstet Gynecol* 1996;**174**:1343–53.

6 Dunne F. Type 2 diabetes in pregnancy. *Semin Fetal Neonatal Med* 2005;**10**:333–40.

7 Penney GC, Mair G, Pearson DW. Scottish diabetes in pregnancy group. Outcomes of pregnancy in women with type 1 diabetes in Scotland; a national population-based study. *BJOG* 2003;**110**:315–8.

8 Naylor CD. Diagnosing gestational diabetes mellitus. Is the gold standard valid? *Diabetes Care* 1989;**12**:565–72.

9 Coustan DR. Gestational diabetes. *Diabetes Care* 1993;**16**(Suppl 3):8–15.

10 Freinkel N. Effects of the conceptus on maternal metabolism during pregnancy. In: Lerbal BS, Wrenshall GA (eds.), *On the Nature and Treatment of Diabetes*. Amsterdam. Excerpt Medica; 1965:679.

11 Dornhorst A, Frost G. The dietary management of diabetic pregnancies. In: Frost G, Dornhorst A, Moses R (eds.), *Nutritional Management of Diabetes Mellitus*. Chichester, UK: John Wiley and Sons Ltd.; 2003.

12 American College of Obstetricians and Gynaecologists: Management of diabetes mellitus in pregnancy. *ACOG Tech Bull* 1986;**92**:1–5.

13 Ray JG, Singh G, Burrows RF. Evidence for suboptimal use of periconceptional folic acid supplements globally. *BJOG* 2004;**111**:399–408.

14 Relton CL, Hammal DM, Rankin J, Parker L. Folic acid supplementation and social deprivation. *Public Health Nutr* 2005;**8**:338–40.

15 Brown CJ, Dawson A, Dodds R, et al. Report of the Pregnancy and Neonatal Care Group. *Diabetic Med* 1996;**13**(9 Suppl 4):543–53.

16 Stiete H, Stiete S, Petschaelis A, et al. Malformations in diabetic pregnancy. *Diabetologia* 1994;**37**(Suppl 1):A172.

17 Crowther C, Hillier J, Moss J, et al. Effect of treatment of gestational diabetes on pregnancy outcomes. *N Engl J Med* 2005;**325**(24):2477–86.

18 Diabetes UK Nutrition Subcommittee of the Diabetes Care Advisory Committee. The implementation of nutritional advice for people with diabetes. *Diabetic Med* 2003;**20**:786–807.

19 Pittendreigh J. Food facts: healthy eating during pregnancy. Birmingham, AL: British Dietetic Association. Available at: http://.www.bda. uk/latest-food-facts.php. Accessed March 2006.

20 Coustan DR, Imrah J. Prophylactic insulin treatment of gestational diabetes reduces the incidence of macrosomia, operative delivery and birth trauma. *Am J Obstet Gynecol* 1984;**150**:836–42.
21 Anderson JH, Jr, Brunelle RL, Koivisto VA, et al. Reduction of postprandial hyperglycaemia and frequency of hypoglycaemia in IDDM patients on insulin-analog treatment. *Diabetes* 1997;**46**:265–70.
22 Pettit DJ, Ospina P, Kolaczynski JW, Jovanovic L. Comparison of an insulin analog, insulin aspart and regular human insulin with no insulin in gestational diabetes mellitus. *Diabetes Care* 2003;**26**: 183–6.
23 Fineberg NS, Fineberg SE, Anderson JH, et al. Immunologic effects of insulin lispro (Lys (B23), Pro (B29) human insulin) in IDDM and NIDDM patients previously treated with insulin. *Diabetes* 1996;**45**:1750–4.
24 Wyatt JW, Frias J, Hoyme E, et al. Congenital anomaly rate in offspring of women with diabetes treated with Humalog. *Diabetologia* 2003;**46**(Suppl 2):A259.
25 Kitzmiller J, Main E, Ward B, Theiss T, Peterson D. Insulin lispro and the development of proliferative diabetic retinopathy during pregnancy. *Diabetes Care* 1999;**22**:874.
26 Langer O, Conway DL, Berkus MD, Xenakis EM, Gonzales O. A comparison of glyburide and insulin in women with gestational diabetes mellitus. *N Engl J Med* 2000;**343**(16):1134–8.
27 Adam PAJ, Schwartz R. Diagnosis and treatment: should oral hypoglycaemic agents be used in paediatric and pregnant patients. *Paediatrics* 1968;**42**:819–23.
28 Coetzee EJ, Jackson WP. Metformin in the management of pregnant non-insulin dependent diabetes. *Diabetologia* 1979;**16**:241–5.
29 Glueck C, Phillips H, Cameron D, et al. Continuing metformin throughout pregnancy in women with polycystic ovary syndrome appears to safely reduce first-trimester spontaneous abortion: a pilot study. *Fertil Steril* 2001;**75**:46–52.
30 Jakubowicz D, Iuorno M, Jakubowicz S, et al. Effects of metformin on early pregnancy in the polycystic ovary syndrome. *J Clin Endocrinol Metab* 2002;**87**:524–9.
31 Glueck C, Wang P, Goldenberg N, Sieve-Smith L. Pregnancy outcomes among women with polycystic ovary syndrome treated with metformin. *Hum Reprod* 2002;**17**:2858–64.
32 Glueck C, Bornovali N, Goldenberg N, et al. Pre-eclampsia, polycystic ovary syndrome, metformin and pregnancy outcomes. *Diabet Med*
33 Glueck C, Wang P, Kobayashi S, et al. Metformin therapy throughout pregnancy reduces the development of gestational diabetes in women with polycystic ovary syndrome. *Fertil Steril* 2002;**77**: 520–5.
34 Gillmer MD, Beard RW, Brooke FM, Oakley NW. Carbohydrate metabolism in pregnancy. Part 1. Diurnal plasma glucose profile in normal and diabetic women. *Br Med J* 1975;**iii**:402–4.

35 Gillmer MD, Holmes SM, Moore MP, et al. Diabetes in pregnancy; obstetric management. In: Sutherland HW, Stowers JM (eds.), *Carbohydrate Metabolism in Pregnancy and the Newborn*. Edinburgh: Churchill Livingstone; 1984:102–18.
36 Hale T, Kristensen J, Hackett L, et al. Transfer of metformin into human milk. *Diabetologia* 2002;**45**:1509–14.

CHAPTER 11
Treatment of asthma

Catherine Williamson, Anita Banerjee

Key points

- Many asthmatic women get worse during pregnancy because they stop taking their medication
- The drug treatment of asthma during pregnancy should be the same as in the non-pregnant women
- Regular inhaled anti-inflammatory medication is first-line maintenance treatment and is safe in pregnancy
- Steroids should be used to treat asthma in pregnancy if clinically indicated
- If chest radiography is clinically indicated, then it should be performed

Introduction

Asthma is by far the most common chronic illness of young adulthood, and all those involved in the care of women during pregnancy and childbirth will encounter asthmatics. Asthma affects 3.0–8.3% of pregnant women around the world and the prevalence is rising [1]. In the UK five deaths related to asthma were reported in the Confidential Enquiry into Maternal Deaths from 2000 to 2002 [2]. This chapter outlines the normal physiological changes in the respiratory system during pregnancy, the interactions between asthma and pregnancy and goes on to deal with the special considerations relating to prescribing for the pregnant woman with asthma.

Prescribing in Pregnancy, 4th edition. Edited by Peter Rubin and Margaret Ramsay,
 ISBN: 978-1-4051-4712-5.

Changes in respiratory function during pregnancy

During pregnancy, oxygen consumption is increased by around 20% and the maternal metabolic rate by about 15%. This additional demand is met by a 40–50% increase in resting minute ventilation, resulting from a rise in tidal volume rather than respiratory rate. This change in ventilation is thought to be due to stimulatory effect of progesterone on ventilatory drive centrally. The maternal hyperventilation leads to a reduction in partial pressure of arterial carbon dioxide ($PaCO_2$) to 4.0 kPa, and there is a compensatory fall in serum bicarbonate to 18–22 mmol/L. A mild respiratory alkalosis is therefore normal in pregnancy, with an arterial pH of 7.44.

During a normal pregnancy up to 75% of women experience a subjective feeling of breathlessness, possibly as a consequence of increased awareness of the physiological hyperventilation. This 'dyspnoea of pregnancy' is most common in the third trimester and may lead to diagnostic confusion. Later in pregnancy, there is a decrease in functional residual capacity when the diaphragmatic position and configuration of the chest wall is altered, but since the diaphragm excursion is unaffected, the vital capacity is unchanged.

The effect of pregnancy on asthma

The effect of pregnancy on asthma has been reviewed by many groups in the past. A meta-analysis reviewing both retrospective and prospective data concluded that in one-third of women asthma improves during pregnancy, in one-third there is no change and in another third asthma worsens [3].

There have been several studies of the gestation at which the asthma is likely to worsen. One group showed that worsening symptoms of asthma did not occur until the fourth month of gestation, and the peak incidence of flares occurred during the sixth month [4]. Another study showed that symptoms of asthma worsened between weeks 29 and 36 [5], while a third group reported exacerbations during weeks 17–24 [6]. Interestingly it has also been shown that asthma, regardless of severity, improves in the last four weeks of pregnancy [7].

It is important to assess the severity of asthma predating the pregnancy, since there is evidence that a woman who had more severe asthma pre-pregnancy will have more exacerbations during the pregnancy [4,5,8]. By the third postpartum month the severity of the asthma tends to return to the pre-pregnancy level, even in those women where the severity of the asthma has changed during pregnancy [9]. Whatever happens to the severity of the disease process itself, many asthmatics experience worsening of their symptoms during pregnancy simply because they have stopped or reduced their usual medications due to fears (their own or those of their doctors) about their safety.

The effect of asthma on pregnancy and its outcome

Most of the prospective and relatively large studies have indicated that women with mild to moderate asthma have good maternal and perinatal outcomes, whereas women requiring oral corticosteroids and stratified as having severe asthma are at significant risk for poor maternal and perinatal outcome.

A recent population-based study including 963 asthmatic women reported favourable perinatal outcomes but found an increase risk for adverse maternal outcome including diabetes mellitus, hypertensive disorders and higher rates of caesarean sections than in the non-asthmatic women [10]. A large multicentre prospective study took into consideration asthma severity and management [11]. It showed that preterm delivery was not associated with asthma diagnosis or severity, but oral corticosteroid use was associated with a reduction in gestation period by 2.22 weeks and theophylline use was associated with a reduction in gestation period by 1.11 weeks. Increasing asthma severity and symptoms were associated with small-for-gestational-age infants.

However, not all studies agree with this finding and an observational study involving 16 centres that stratified patients according to asthma severity found no significant differences in the rates of preterm delivery, gestational diabetes, pre-eclampsia, preterm labour, small-for-gestational-age infants, chorioamnionitis, oligohydramnios and congenital malformations. This study did demonstrate increased caesarean section rates in the moderate to severe asthmatic group [12]. In secondary analysis they found that during the course of the pregnancy 23.0% had an improvement in asthma severity and 30.3% had a worsening in asthma severity [8]. In 2006 a review of all the past studies of asthma in pregnancy concluded that those populations with mild to moderate asthma have good maternal and perinatal outcomes, whereas women requiring oral corticosteroids and stratified as having severe asthma are at significant risk for poor maternal and perinatal outcome [13].

Management of asthma in pregnancy

Much unnecessary impairment of quality of life results from failure to diagnose or adequately treat asthma. Since virtually all women are under some form of medical supervision during pregnancy, this is an ideal time to recognize undiagnosed asthma and to achieve optimum disease control in women known to be asthmatic [14]. It is important to offer women pre-pregnancy counselling regarding the importance of continuing their asthma medication during pregnancy to ensure good asthma control and to advise those who smoke regarding the dangers of smoking for themselves and their baby and then giving appropriate support to stop smoking.

The successful management of asthma during pregnancy requires a multidisciplinary approach, involving the obstetrician, the respiratory physician, the asthma nurse and the woman. The emphasis is on prevention and not on exacerbations of asthma alone. Asthma exacerbations lead to increasing morbidity and mortality, and asthma in pregnancy should be treated as for non-pregnant women. Pregnant women with asthma should be monitored closely during pregnancy and any change in the course of the disease should be matched with an appropriate change in therapy. Regular, inhaled anti-inflammatory medication is the mainstay of maintenance treatment for all those with infrequent symptoms (less than once daily). A stepwise approach to asthma medication is essential to control symptoms: steroid inhalers followed by long-acting inhaled β_2-agonists. Systemic steroids are to be used when indicated. Leukotriene antagonists should not be commenced during pregnancy, but they be may continued if a woman has demonstrated, prior to pregnancy, significant improvement not achievable with other medications [15].

Patient education and home peak flow monitoring with personalised self-management plans have been shown to reduce the morbidity in asthmatics [16–18]. Peak flow meters can be prescribed to help women to monitor their asthma throughout pregnancy.

Drug treatment

The drug treatment of asthma in pregnancy is no different from that in non-pregnant women. Most drugs used to treat asthma

Table 11.1 The safety of drugs that can be used for the treatment of asthma in pregnancy

Drug	First trimester	Second trimester	Third trimester
Inhaled/nebulised short-acting β_2-agonists	Safe	Safe	Safe
Inhaled corticosteroids	Safe	Safe	Safe
Oral corticosteroids	Small risk of cleft palate	Safe	Safe
Inhaled long-acting β_2-agonists	Safe	Safe	Safe
Theophyllines	Safe	Safe	Safe
Inhaled cromoglycate	Safe	Safe	Safe
Anticholinergics	Safe	Safe	Safe
Leukotriene antagonists	Unsure	Unsure	Unsure

appear safe (Table 11.1). Considerations concerning individual treatments are discussed below. Table 11.2 summarizes the major studies of the pregnancy outcome of women who were taking specific drugs to treat asthma in pregnancy. Only studies with a control group are included.

Systemic corticosteroids

Prednisolone is metabolised by the placenta and very little (10%) active drug ever reaches the fetus. On administering large doses of corticosteroids to pregnant mice, rats and rabbits during organogenesis, the offspring were born with cleft palate [26–28]. Subsequent human studies found little evidence of poor maternal and fetal outcome associated with corticosteroid use, and a meta-analysis of six cohort studies in which corticosteroids were used in the first trimester showed there was no increased risk of total congenital malformations [19,29,30]. However, this meta-analysis did suggest that there is increased risk of oral clefts (odds ratio (OR), 3.35; 95% CI, 1.97–5.69) [31].

Systemic steroids have serious and well-known side effects when given frequently or in high doses for prolonged periods. Women and their doctors may be reluctant to use these drugs in pregnancy, and their concerns extend to the use of inhaled corticosteroids. This concern is misplaced and steroids should be used to treat asthma in pregnancy in the same way as in the non-pregnant asthmatic women. A prospective cohort study of 51 pregnant women with

Table 11.2 Complications of asthma medication in pregnancy

Drug	No. of cases	Congenital malformations	Other adverse outcomes	References
Inhaled short-acting bronchodilators	259	Not increased*	Not increased*	[9]
	488	Not increased*	Not increased*	[19]
	1753	Not increased*	Not increased*	[20]
Inhaled corticosteroids	2968	Not reported	Slight increased LBW†	[21]
	2014	Not increased†	Not reported*	[22]
	89	Not increased*	Not increased*	[19]
Oral corticosteroids	130	Not reported	Increased pre-eclampsia*	[19]
	58	Not reported	Increased pre-eclampsia*	[23]
	31	Not increased*	Increased LBW, prematurity and maternal impaired glucose tolerance*	[11]
	185	Not increased	Increased LBW and preterm delivery*	[20]
Inhaled long-acting bronchodilators	93	Not increased†	Not reported	[19]
	64	Not reported	Not increased*	[11]
Theophyllines	212	Not increased*	Increased pre-eclampsia and neonatal jaundice*	[24]
	273	Not increased*	Not increased*	[20]
Cromoglycate	243	Not increased*	Not increased*	[19]

This table summarizes the major studies in which the pregnancy outcome in women who were taking specific drugs for asthma was compared with that of controls.

*Compared with an unexposed control group; †compared with the general population. LBW, low birth weight.

Adapted from Chambers [25] and Schatz et al. [19].

an exacerbation of asthma found that compared to non-pregnant women they were equally likely to be admitted from an accident and emergency setting; but they were less likely to be prescribed corticosteroids if sent home. At 2-week follow-up the pregnant women were 2.9 times more likely to report symptoms of an ongoing exacerbation of asthma [32]. Short courses of oral steroids are required for acute exacerbations of asthma that fail to respond to an increased dose of inhaled steroids. Rarely, a patient with severe asthma may require long-term maintenance oral steroids. Such individuals will take inhaled steroids to minimise the oral dose requirements and the risk of the systemic side effects.

Pre-eclampsia, gestational diabetes, low birth weight and preterm delivery have all been associated with systemic corticosteroid use during pregnancy [19,23,32–35]. One case control study of 81 pregnant asthmatics, included 31 steroid-dependent individuals, and 130 pregnant controls found that steroid-dependent asthmatics were at significantly increased risk for gestational (12.90% versus 1.59%) and insulin-requiring diabetes (9.7% versus 0.0%). Preterm delivery and low birth weight were complications observed significantly more often in the steroid-dependent asthmatics when compared to the non-steroid-medication-dependent asthmatics (54.8% versus 14.0% and 45.2% versus 14.0%, respectively) [35]. In a prospective study of 824 asthmatic women and 678 non-asthmatic women, a multivariate analysis found oral corticosteroids were independently associated with pre-eclampsia (OR, 2.0; 95% CI, 1.11–3.61; $p = 0.027$) [19]. However, another multicentre observational study involving 881 non-asthmatics, 873 with mild asthma, 814 with moderate and 52 with severe asthma found no significant differences for maternal complications except for an increase in overall caesarean delivery rate among the moderate or severe asthmatic group (OR, 1.4; 95% CI, 1.1–1.8) [36]. In summary, these studies indicate that severe asthma is associated with worsening outcomes. However, it is difficult to ascertain whether this is the result of the underlying severity of the disease or the requirement for corticosteroid treatment. On balance, a review of the potential risks and benefits indicates that corticosteroids are indicated in the treatment of asthma.

Although suppression of the fetal hypothalamic-pituitary-adrenal axis is a theoretical possibility when the mother is treated with systemic steroids, there is no evidence from clinical practice to support this. Further reassurance comes from a study in which the adrenocortical reserve of six newborns whose mothers had received long-term systemic steroids was formally assessed, and the response to exogenous adrenocorticotrophic hormone was normal [37]. Maternal adrenal insufficiency is, however, a possibility, and if the woman has been taking more than 7.5 mg of prednisolone for 2 weeks or more, the authors agree that accepted practice would include the administration of parenteral steroids (hydrocortisone 100 mg three times a day) to cover the stress of labour and delivery.

Prolonged use of oral steroids increases the risk of gestational diabetes and causes deterioration in blood glucose control in those women with established impairment of glucose tolerance in pregnancy. Provided clinicians are aware of this and check the blood glucose regularly, the hyperglycaemia is amenable to treatment with diet and, if required, insulin; this is reversible once the steroid dose is stopped or reduced. The development of hyperglycaemia is not, however, an indication to discontinue or decrease the dose of oral steroids, the requirements for which must be determined by the asthma.

The rare, but important, psychiatric side effects of oral glucocorticoids should be remembered, and all women who have been commenced on steroids should be reviewed within 1 week.

Inhaled corticosteroids

Inhaled steroids are known to prevent exacerbations of asthma in the non-pregnant state. No harm to the fetus from inhaled steroids has been shown. Furthermore, only minimum amounts of inhaled corticosteroid preparations are systemically absorbed [22]. This should be emphasised, as decreasing or stopping treatment with inhaled anti-inflammatory drugs during pregnancy often causes a potentially dangerous deterioration in disease control. Indeed, one study has found a higher incidence of asthma exacerbations in those who were not treated initially with inhaled corticosteroid in comparison with those who had been on inhaled steroids from the beginning of pregnancy [6]. A randomised double-blind study has given further support to the efficacy of inhaled steroids during pregnancy. In this study, inhaled beclomethasone dipropionate was compared with oral theophylline for the prevention of acute exacerbations of asthma in pregnancy and there was no significant difference in the frequency of exacerbations, but fewer side effects were reported in the steroid inhaler arm [36]. The population-based Swedish Medical Birth Register cohort study found no added risk for major congenital malformations in 2014 infants born to asthmatic women using the inhaled steroid budesonide [21]. The same register found no increased risk of low birth weight, stillbirth and preterm delivery in 2968 budesonide-exposed pregnancies [38].

A randomised, double-blind, placebo control study including 319 pregnancies found no difference in outcome regarding miscarriages, congenital malformations and other outcomes when comparing mild to moderate persistent asthmatics receiving low-dose budesonide to placebo [39]. A nested case control study found no increased risk of pregnancy-induced hypertension (OR, 1.02; 95% CI, 0.77–1.34) or pre-eclampsia (OR, 1.06; 95% CI, 0.74–1.53) amongst users of inhaled corticosteroids during pregnancy [40].

Examples of the available steroid inhalers include beclomethasone (Becotide, Beclazone, Qvar), budesonide (Pulmicort), fluticasone (Flixotide), mometasone (Asmanex). There are no data to suggest that other more new inhaled corticosteroids are less safe in pregnancy and though the preferred inhaled steroid is budesonide if the woman is well controlled with regards to her asthma before pregnancy with any of the alternative corticosteroid inhalers, it would be reasonable to continue with that inhaler, since non-compliance may be more detrimental. Use of a spacer device when inhaled steroids need to be administered will reduce oropharyngeal candidiasis, improve delivery of the drug and decrease the possibility of systemic effects.

In summary, inhaled, nebulised, oral and parenteral corticosteroids may need to be used in pregnancy. Maternal and fetal outcome is far more affected by non-compliance or reluctance to step up corticosteroid treatment.

β_2-Agonists

Inhaled β_2-agonists such as salbutamol and terbutaline provide rapid and effective relief of bronchospasm. Tremor and tachycardia are the most common dose-related side effects of these drugs. Maternal pulmonary oedema, hypokalaemia and hyperglycaemia are potential but rare adverse effects when high-dose β_2-agonists are given intravenously to treat acute severe asthma and preterm labour.

Transfer of β_2-agonists from the systemic circulation across the placenta is relatively rapid, but very little of a given inhaled dose reaches the lungs and only a minute fraction of this reaches the systemic circulation. Studies have looked specifically at perinatal outcomes and major congenital malformations. In a study of 401 women exposed to short-acting ß$_2$-agonists, no significant increase for preterm labour or increased low birth weight was found [11,20,41]. A prospective study of 488 pregnant women exposed to ß$_2$-agonists compared to non-asthmatic pregnant women found no increased risk of major congenital abnormalities or other perinatal outcomes [20]. A larger study of 1753 pregnant women exposed to ß$_2$-agonists showed no increased risk for preterm labour, gestational hypertension, low birth weight, pre-eclampsia or major congenital abnormalities [41].

Two long-acting inhaled bronchodilators are available, salmeterol and formoterol. There are few studies looking at maternal and fetal outcomes in these agents. In one study where there were 91 pregnancy exposures to salmeterol in the first trimester, the rates of congenital anomalies, spontaneous abortion and preterm labour were equivalent to the general population [42]. Another small study of 31 women exposed to formoterol reported that 8% of infants had major congenital malformations. However, extrapolation from these findings is difficult due to the small numbers of cases exposed to formoterol [43]. Although there is less information regarding their safety than for older treatments, we would not discontinue their use in a woman with labile asthma who is stable on these drugs during pregnancy.

Disodium cromoglycate and nedocromil

Inhaled cromoglycate is generally more widely used in the management of asthma in children than in adults. A study of 243 first-trimester-exposed women found it to be safe for both mother and fetus [19]. Nedocromil is a more recently introduced preparation with a pharmacological action similar to sodium cromoglycate. However, at the present time there are no data about its safety in pregnancy.

Methylxanthines

These drugs are no longer used as first-line therapy for asthma. A modified-release oral preparation may be added to conventional therapy with inhaled bronchodilators and inhaled corticosteroids, especially to control night-time symptoms and wheeze. Both theophylline and aminophylline readily cross the placenta and fetal theophylline levels are similar to those of the mother

[44]. Although theophylline has been shown to be a potent cardiovascular teratogen in animals, there is no conclusive evidence of congenital malformations in the human fetus [15,45–47]. A prospective study found no increase in major congenital malformations in 429 women who took theophylline in pregnancy, of which 68% were exposed to the drug in the first trimester [19]. A case control study of 212 theophylline treated asthmatics, 292 pregnant asthmatics without theophylline and 237 controls found no significant risks for major congenital malformations. However, the frequency of neonatal jaundice necessitating treatment doubled in the theophylline-treated arm, which may be explained by a trend to higher rates of prematurity in this group and the fact that the theophylline-treated group were treated for more exacerbations of asthma [46].

Pharmacokinetic data concerning xanthines in pregnancy are conflicting. The increased blood volumes associated with pregnancy may lead to lower concentrations of active drug. In contrast, a small study suggested a 20–30% reduction of theophylline clearance in the third trimester, but this has not been confirmed by more recent studies [24,48,49]. Some have noted transient tachycardia or irritability in neonates of mothers receiving xanthines, but others found mean neonatal heart rate and Apgar scores were unaffected by maternal use of theophylline [44].

Anticholinergic drugs

Anticholinergic drugs have traditionally been considered more effective in the management of chronic bronchitis than asthma, but inhaled ipratropium bromide can be added if symptoms are not optimally controlled with regular corticosteroid and $ß_2$-agonists. No adverse fetal affects have been reported but, as with atropine, there may be a minimal increase in fetal heart rate.

Leukotriene antagonists

Leukotrienes are metabolites of arachidonic acid which act as mediators of inflammation and cause smooth muscle contraction and proliferation. The leukotriene antagonist montelukast is currently licensed in the UK as monotherapy for the prophylaxis of exercise-induced asthma in patients aged 6 years and older. Zafirlukast is licensed in patients older than 12 years and can be used as first-line therapy instead of inhaled corticosteroids. A pregnancy registry is being maintained for montelukast by Merck Research Laboratories and this contains data on 151 prospective pregnancies. To date there have been 116 first-trimester exposures and 7 major congenital malformations [50]. There still remains insufficient information to establish whether leukotriene antagonists are safe in pregnancy.

Management of acute severe asthma

Acute severe attacks of asthma are life-threatening and should be managed in the hospital setting. The treatment is no different from the emergency management of acute severe asthma in the non-pregnant state. Oxygen, nebulised bronchodilators, oral or intravenous steroids and, in severe cases, magnesium sulphate, intravenous aminophylline or intravenous β_2-agonists should be used as indicated. A single dose of magnesium sulphate is used in acute severe asthma; 1.2–2.0 g is given intravenously over 20 minutes. The dose of magnesium sulphate used for the prevention of eclampsia [51] is higher than that used for the treatment of asthma. Therefore, given the wide experience of its use in pregnancy, it is unlikely to be associated with adverse fetal outcomes when used in late pregnancy. Data relating to first-trimester magnesium sulphate treatment are more limited.

The ionising radiation from a chest X-ray is approximately 0.2 rad (less than 1/20th of the maximum recommended exposure in pregnancy which is 5.0 rad) and abdominal shielding will minimize the exposure to the fetus. If a chest X-ray is clinically indicated, this investigation must not be withheld just because the patient is pregnant.

Other considerations when prescribing for the pregnant asthmatic

Aspirin

Low-dose aspirin is used as prophylaxis for certain women at very high risk of early onset pre-eclampsia, but it is worth remembering that some asthmatics are allergic to aspirin [52]. The prevalence of aspirin sensitivity in pregnant asthmatic was reported as 15% in a study of 504 patients [46]. Therefore it is important to ask about a history of such sensitivity before treatment is started with low-dose aspirin.

Management of respiratory infection

Upper and lower respiratory tract infections (bacterial and viral) are common precipitants for deterioration in asthma. The production of yellow or green sputum is not diagnostic of a lower respiratory tract infection and may indicate an exacerbation of asthma with eosinophils in the sputum. However, if there are other pointers to infection (e.g., fever, chest signs), antibiotics should be prescribed.

The antibiotics most frequently used in respiratory infections, including the penicillins, cephalosporins and macrolides, are safe in pregnancy. Amoxicillin should be given in higher than usual dosage (500 mg 8-hourly) in pregnancy, because of increased renal clearance. Tetracycline causes permanent staining of the child's teeth, has adverse effects on the fetal skeleton and is contraindicated in pregnancy, with rare exceptions where the health of the mother takes precedence over the risk to the fetus. Similarly, cough medicines containing iodine are contraindicated since the iodine is taken up by the fetal thyroid and may cause hypothyroidism and fetal goitre.

Adults in general and pregnant women in particular are susceptible to varicella zoster (chickenpox) pneumonia and the maternal and fetal mortality is high [53]. Because of the substantial risk to the mother, non-immune pregnant women exposed to varicella should be given zoster-immune globulin [54]. Patients taking systemic corticosteroids are at especially high risk of severe varicella, and it has been suggested that patients should be asked about a previous history of varicella prior to commencing steroids [55]. If the history is doubtful, antibody status should be checked and those who are found to be seronegative must be told to attend immediately and receive prophylaxis with zoster-immune globulin following inadvertent exposure to varicella.

Management during labour and delivery

Although they are the most common fears of asthmatic women entering pregnancy, acute attacks of asthma during labour and delivery are extremely rare, and women should be reassured accordingly. The explanation for this rarity is uncertain, although it is possible that it is related to an increase in endogenous corticosteroids or catecholamine production at this time. Women should continue their regular inhalers throughout their labour, and those on maintenance oral steroids (>7.5 mg prednisolone daily) or being treated with steroids for more than 2 weeks before the onset of labour or delivery should receive parenteral steroids during labour, and until they are able to restart their own medication. Prostaglandin E_2 used to induce labour, to ripen the cervix or for early termination of pregnancy is a bronchodilator and is safe to use. Prostaglandin $F_{2\alpha}$ carboprost, used in the emergency management of postpartum haemorrhage, may cause bronchospasm, especially in conjunction with general anaesthesia [56,57].

All forms of pain relief in labour, including epidural analgesia and Entonox, may be safely used by asthmatic women, although opiates should be avoided in the unlikely event of an acute asthmatic attack. If anaesthesia is required, women should be encouraged to have an epidural rather than general anaesthesia because of the increased risk of chest infection and associated atelectasis in people with asthma. Although ergometrine has been reported to cause bronchospasm, particularly in association with general anaesthesia, this does not seem to be a practical problem when Syntometrine (oxytocin + ergometrine) is used to prevent postpartum haemorrhage.

NSAIDS are commonly used for pain relief post-caesarean section. Women with asthma should be asked about any known aspirin or NSAID allergy, prior to the use of these drugs. If a woman has such a history, it is safer to use an alternative form of analgesia.

Breastfeeding

Women with asthma should be encouraged to breastfeed their babies if they wish, due to the nutritional, immunological and psychological benefits. The risk of atopic disease developing in the child of an asthmatic woman is about one in ten, or one in three if both parents are atopic.

There is evidence that the risk of atopic diseases may be reduced by breastfeeding [58]. A 15-year prospective study has shown that breastfeeding and delaying exposure to allergens reduce the frequency of clinical allergic disease, and prolonged breastfeeding may lower the incidence of severe or obvious atopic disease, particularly in babies with a family history of atopy [59,60]. However, controversy arose when a prospective longitudinal study of 1246 newborns found exclusive breastfeeding was associated with a significantly lower rate of wheezing in the first 2 years of life irrespective of maternal asthma (OR, 0.45; 95% CI, 0.2–0.9) but after 6 years of age exclusive breastfeeding was related to a higher rate of asthma in atopic children of mothers with asthma (OR, 5.7; 95% CI, 2.3–14.1) [61]. In contrast, a 6-year follow-up of 2602 infants found no correlation between maternal asthma and the development of subsequent asthma in the breastfed children [62]. Therefore we believe that breastfeeding should still be advocated in asthmatic women regardless of the fact that the above data are conflicting, since there are overall benefits to mother and child.

All the drugs employed in the management of asthma, including oral steroids, are safe to use when breastfeeding. Small amounts of prednisolone and prednisone are secreted in breast milk, and, although continuous maternal use of high-dose corticosteroids could theoretically affect the infant's adrenal function, this is unlikely with doses below 30 mg prednisolone per day [63,64]. No clinical side effects have been reported in infants breastfed by mothers receiving prednisolone. A small study examining the secretion of tritium-labelled prednisolone in breast milk showed that a mean of only 0.14% of radioactivity from an oral dose of 5 mg of prednisolone was recovered per litre of breast milk [63].

Theophylline appears in breast milk, with milk-to-plasma ratio of 0.7, reaching a peak concentration 2 hours after peak plasma levels [65]. We are not aware of any reports of significant problems in clinical practice resulting from transfer of methylxanthines in breast milk, and the proportion of new mothers who need methylxanthines is small.

Conclusion

Management of asthma in pregnancy does not differ significantly from management in the non-pregnant state. The priority should be effective control of the disease process, with the aim of having total freedom from symptoms both day and night. More attention must, however, be given to explanation and reassurance about the safety of the drugs used to treat asthma during pregnancy and lactation.

The risk of harm to the fetus comes from poorly controlled asthma rather than from the drugs used to prevent or treat asthma. Good control of asthma sets a pattern for future management; the mother–infant relationship may not flourish in the presence of chronic maternal ill health. Asthma in pregnancy should be regarded as an opportunity to gain long-term benefit, not just as a challenge lasting 9 months.

Acknowledgements

The authors would like to acknowledge Dr Catherine Nelson-Piercy, author of this chapter in previous editions of this book, for her substantial contribution.

References

1 Kwon HL, Belanger K, Bracken MB. Asthma prevalence among pregnant and childbearing-aged women in the United States: estimates from national health surveys. *Ann Epidemiol* 2003;**13**:317–24.

2 Department of Health Welsh Office, Scottish Home Heath Department and Department of Health and Social Services Northern Ireland. Confidential enquiries into maternal deaths in the United Kingdom 2000–2002. London: HMSO; 2005.

3 Juniper EF, Newhouse MT. Effect of pregnancy on asthma: a systematic review and metaanalysis. In: Schatz M, Zeiger RS, Claman HN (eds.), *Asthma and Immunological Diseases in Pregnancy and Early Infancy.* New York: Marcel Dekker; 1993:223–50.

4 Gluck JC, Gluck P. The effects of pregnancy on asthma: a prospective study. *Ann Allergy* 1976;**37**:164–8.

5 Schatz M, Harden K, Forsythe A, et al. The course of asthma during pregnancy, post partum, and with successive pregnancies: a prospective analysis. *J Allergy Clin Immunol* 1988;**81**:509–17.

6 Stenius-Aarniala BS, Hedman J, Teramo KA. Acute asthma during pregnancy. *Thorax* 1996;**51**:411–4.

7 White RJ, Coutts II, Gibbs CJ, MacIntyre C. A prospective study of asthma during pregnancy and the puerperium. *Respir Med* 1989;**83**:103–6.

8 Schatz M, Dombrowski MP, Wise R, et al. Asthma morbidity during pregnancy can be predicted by severity classification. *J Allergy Clin Immunol* 2003;**112**:283–8.

9 Schatz M, Zeiger RS, Harden KM, et al. The safety of inhaled beta-agonist bronchodilators during pregnancy. *J Allergy Clin Immunol* 1988;**82**:686–95.

10 Sheiner E, Mazor M, Levy A, Wiznitzer A, Bashiri A. Pregnancy outcome of asthmatic patients: a population-based study. *J Matern Fetal Neonatal Med* 2005;**18**:237–40.

11 Bracken MB, Triche EW, Belanger K, Saftlas A, Beckett WS, Leaderer BP. Asthma symptoms, severity, and drug therapy: a prospective study of effects on 2205 pregnancies. *Obstet Gynecol* 2003;**102**:739–52.

12 Dombrowski MP, Schatz M, Wise R, et al. Asthma during pregnancy. *Obstet Gynecol* 2004;**103**:5–12.

13 Dombrowski MP. Outcomes of pregnancy in asthmatic women. *Immunol Allergy Clin North Am* 2006;**26**:81–92.

14 Moore-Gillon J. Asthma in pregnancy. *Br J Obstet Gynaecol* 1994; **101**:658–60.
15 Asthma in adults and schoolchildren. The General Practitioner in Asthma Group, the British Association of Accident and Emergency Medicine, the British Paediatric Respiratory Society and the Royal College of Paediatrics and Child Health. *Thorax* 1997;**52(**Suppl 1):S2–5, S20.
16 Beasley R, Cushley M, Holgate ST. A self management plan in the treatment of adult asthma. *Thorax* 1989;**44**:200–4.
17 Charlton I, Charlton G, Broomfield J, Mullee MA. Evaluation of peak flow and symptoms only self management plans for control of asthma in general practice. *BMJ* 1990;**301**:1355–9.
18 Murphy VE, Gibson PG, Talbot PI, Kessell CG, Clifton VL. Asthma self-management skills and the use of asthma education during pregnancy. *Eur Respir J* 2005;**26**:435–41.
19 Schatz M, Zeiger RS, Harden K, Hoffman CC, Chilingar L, Petitti D. The safety of asthma and allergy medications during pregnancy. *J Allergy Clin Immunol* 1997;**100**:301–6.
20 Schatz M. Asthma treatment during pregnancy. What can be safely taken? *Drug Saf* 1997;**16**:342–50.
21 Kallen B, Rydhstroem H, Aberg A. Congenital malformations after the use of inhaled budesonide in early pregnancy. *Obstet Gynecol* 1999;**93**: 392–5.
22 Harris DM. Some properties of beclomethasone dipropionate and related steroids in man. *Postgrad Med J* 1975;**51**(Suppl 4):20–5.
23 Stenius-Aarniala B, Piirila P, Teramo K. Asthma and pregnancy: a prospective study of 198 pregnancies. *Thorax* 1988;**43**:12–18.
24 Carter BL, Driscoll CE, Smith GD. Theophylline clearance during pregnancy. *Obstet Gynecol* 1986;**68**:555–9.
25 Chambers C. Safety of asthma and allergy medications in pregnancy. *Immunol Allergy Clin North Am* 2006;**26**:13–28.
26 Fainstat T. Cortisone-induced congenital cleft palate in rabbits. *Endocrinology* 1954;**55**:502–8.
27 Pinsky L, Digeorge AM. Cleft palate in the mouse: a teratogenic index of glucocorticoid potency. *Science* 1965;**147**:402–3.
28 Walker BE. Induction of cleft palate in rats with antiinflammatory drugs. *Teratology* 1971;**4**:39–42.
29 Fitzsimons R, Greenberger PA, Patterson R. Outcome of pregnancy in women requiring corticosteroids for severe asthma. *J Allergy Clin Immunol* 1986;**78**:349–53.
30 Schatz M, Patterson R, Zeitz S, O'Rourke J, Melam H. Corticosteroid therapy for the pregnant asthmatic patient. *JAMA* 1975;**233**:804–7.
31 Park-Wyllie L, Mazzotta P, Pastuszak A, et al. Birth defects after maternal exposure to corticosteroids: prospective cohort study and meta-analysis of epidemiological studies. *Teratology* 2000;**62**:385–92.

32 Cydulka RK, Emerman CL, Schreiber D, Molander KH, Woodruff PG, Camargo CA, Jr. Acute asthma among pregnant women presenting to the emergency department. *Am J Respir Crit Care Med* 1999;**160**:887–92.

33 Bakhireva LN, Jones KL, Schatz M, Johnson D, Chambers CD. Asthma medication use in pregnancy and fetal growth. *J Allergy Clin Immunol* 2005;**116**:503–9.

34 Jana N, Vasishta K, Saha SC, Khunnu B. Effect of bronchial asthma on the course of pregnancy, labour and perinatal outcome. *J Obstet Gynaecol* 1995;**21**:227–32.

35 Perlow JH, Montgomery D, Morgan MA, Towers CV, Porto M. Severity of asthma and perinatal outcome. *Am J Obstet Gynecol* 1992;**167**: 963–7.

36 Dombrowski MP, Schatz M, Wise R, et al. Randomized trial of inhaled beclomethasone dipropionate versus theophylline for moderate asthma during pregnancy. *Am J Obstet Gynecol* 2004;**190**:737–44.

37 Arad I, Landau H. Adrenocortical reserve of neonates born of long-term, steroid-treated mothers. *Eur J Pediatr* 1984;**142**:279–80.

38 Norjavaara E, de Verdier MG. Normal pregnancy outcomes in a population-based study including 2968 pregnant women exposed to budesonide. *J Allergy Clin Immunol* 2003;**111**:736–42.

39 Silverman M, Sheffer A, Diaz PV, et al. Outcome of pregnancy in a randomized controlled study of patients with asthma exposed to budesonide. *Ann Allergy Asthma Immunol* 2005;**95**:566–70.

40 Martel MJ, Rey E, Beauchesne MF, et al. Use of inhaled corticosteroids during pregnancy and risk of pregnancy induced hypertension: nested case-control study. *BMJ* 2005;**330**:230.

41 Schatz M, Dombrowski MP, Wise R, et al. The relationship of asthma medication use to perinatal outcomes. *J Allergy Clin Immunol* 2004;**113**: 1040–5.

42 Wilton LV, Pearce GL, Martin RM, Mackay FJ, Mann RD. The outcomes of pregnancy in women exposed to newly marketed drugs in general practice in England. *Br J Obstet Gynaecol* 1998;**105**:882–9.

43 Wilton LV, Shakir SA. A post-marketing surveillance study of formoterol (Foradil): its use in general practice in England. *Drug Saf* 2002;**25**:213–23.

44 Labovitz E, Spector S. Placental theophylline transfer in pregnant asthmatics. *JAMA* 1982;**247**:786–8.

45 Greenberger P, Patterson R. Safety of therapy for allergic symptoms during pregnancy. *Ann Intern Med* 1978;**89**:234–7.

46 Stenius-Aarniala B, Riikonen S, Teramo K. Slow-release theophylline in pregnant asthmatics. *Chest* 1995;**107**:642–7.

47 Heinonen DP SDSS. *Birth Defects and Drugs in Pregnancy*. Littleton, MA: Publishing Sciences Group; 1977.

48 Frederiksen MC, Ruo TI, Chow MJ, Atkinson AJ, Jr. Theophylline pharmacokinetics in pregnancy. *Clin Pharmacol Ther* 1986;**40**:321–8.

49 Gardner MJ, Schatz M, Cousins L, Zeiger R, Middleton E, Jusko WJ. Longitudinal effects of pregnancy on the pharmacokinetics of theophylline. *Eur J Clin Pharmacol* 1987;**32**:289–95.
50 Merck Research laboratories. Sixth annual report on exposure during pregnancy from the Merck Pregnancy Registry for Singulair covering the period from February 20, 1889 through July, 2005. West Point, PA: Merck Research Labs; 2005.
51 Altman D, Carroli G, Duley L, et al. Do women with pre-eclampsia, and their babies, benefit from magnesium sulphate? The Magpie Trial: a randomised placebo-controlled trial. *Lancet* 2002;**359**:1877–90.
52 CLASP: A randomised trial of low-dose aspirin for the prevention and treatment of pre-eclampsia among 9364 pregnant women. CLASP (Collaborative Low-dose Aspirin Study in Pregnancy) Collaborative Group. *Lancet* 1994;**343**:619–29.
53 Broussard RC, Payne DK, George RB. Treatment with acyclovir of varicella pneumonia in pregnancy. *Chest* 1991;**99**:1045–7.
54 Paryani SG, Arvin AM. Intrauterine infection with varicella-zoster virus after maternal varicella. *N Engl J Med* 1986;**314**:1542–6.
55 Rice P, Simmons K, Carr R, Banatvala J. Near fatal chickenpox during prednisolone treatment. *BMJ* 1994;**309**:1069–70.
56 Fishburne JI, Jr, Brenner WE, Braaksma JT, Hendricks CH. Bronchospasm complicating intravenous prostaglandin F 2a for therapeutic abortion. *Obstet Gynecol* 1972;**39**:892–6.
57 Hyman AL, Spannhake EW, Kadowitz PJ. Prostaglandins and the lung. *Am Rev Respir Dis* 1978;**117**:111–36.
58 van Odijk J, Kull I, Borres MP, et al. Breastfeeding and allergic disease: a multidisciplinary review of the literature (1966–2001) on the mode of early feeding in infancy and its impact on later atopic manifestations. *Allergy* 2003;**58**:833–43.
59 Gruskay FL. Comparison of breast, cow, and soy feedings in the prevention of onset of allergic disease: a 15-year prospective study. *Clin Pediatr (Phila)* 1982;**21**:486–91.
60 Saarinen UM, Kajosaari M, Backman A, Siimes MA. Prolonged breastfeeding as prophylaxis for atopic disease. *Lancet* 1979;**2**:163–6.
61 Wright AL, Holberg CJ, Taussig LM, Martinez FD. Factors influencing the relation of infant feeding to asthma and recurrent wheeze in childhood. *Thorax* 2001;**56**:192–7.
62 Oddy WH, Peat JK, de Klerk NH. Maternal asthma, infant feeding, and the risk of asthma in childhood. *J Allergy Clin Immunol* 2002;**110**:65–7.
63 Katz FH, Duncan BR. Letter: entry of prednisone into human milk. *N Engl J Med* 1975;**293**:1154.
64 McKenzie SA, Selley JA, Agnew JE. Secretion of prednisolone into breast milk. *Arch Dis Child* 1975;**50**:894–6.
65 Yurchak AM, Jusko WJ. Theophylline secretion into breast milk. *Pediatrics* 1976;**57**:518–20.

CHAPTER 12

Drugs of misuse

Mary Hepburn

Introduction

Problem drug use among women of childbearing age increased by almost 500% in the 20 years to the mid-1990s [1] with a consequent increase in drug use by pregnant women. Patterns change with time and vary from area to area, with polydrug use being increasingly common. Use of cannabis is widespread throughout the UK and is not confined to those who have a drug problem. In England in 1995 amongst those seeking treatment for drug problems [2], 80% of female users were aged 15–34 years. Opiate/opioid use was most common, reported as the main or subsidiary drug by more than 90% of those attending for treatment of drug problem (64% heroin, 30% methadone and 6% 'other opiates') and as the main drug of use by more than two-thirds. Amphetamines were next most commonly reported, but this nevertheless represents an underestimate of use. Benzodiazepines as main drug of choice were less common but awareness of illicit benzodiazepine use particularly with opiates/opioids has been steadily increasing [3,4]. In Scotland opiate/opioid use was similarly most commonly reported [5] with heroin followed by methadone as the main drug of use. Use of benzodiazepines by injection was a major problem in Scotland and particularly Glasgow [6], and the injection in combination with opiates/opioids was considered an important factor in drug deaths. A third of those seeking help were women of whom over 90% were aged 15–34 years. Overall in the UK more than a third of those seeking treatment were currently injecting their drugs. The route of use has obvious implications for the severity of effects on pregnancy. Since the turn

Prescribing in Pregnancy, 4th edition. Edited by Peter Rubin and Margaret Ramsay,
 ISBN: 978-1-4051-4712-5.

of the century the relative patterns of reported drug use in the different parts of the UK are largely unchanged with the exception of an increase in the reported use of cocaine, more so in England than in Scotland or Wales. In Scotland diazepam is now the most commonly used benzodiazepine. There has been a reduction in injecting drug use to two-fifths in the UK overall, with the highest rate (40%) in England and the lowest rate (29%) in Wales. The male-to-female ratio is higher in England at 3.1 (www.dh.gov.uk/PublicationsAndStatistics) compared to 2.1 in Scotland (www.drugmisuse.isdScotland.org). Recent Scottish statistics show a gradual trend towards an overall older age profile [7].

Problem drug use occurs more frequently in association with socioeconomic deprivation and the poorer pregnancy outcomes are multifactorial. Identifying the precise effects of the drug use quantitatively or qualitatively can therefore be difficult.

Conception

Heroin has been claimed to cause increased levels of circulating gonadotrophins with an increased incidence of multiple pregnancies [8] but more commonly, it is reported to cause reduced gonadotrophin production, secondary amenorrhoea [9,10] and consequently infertility. While amenorrhoea is common among heroin users, it is important to be aware that this may occur with or without anovulation, so for those who do not want to conceive, adequate contraception is essential.

Use in pregnancy

General effects on mother and baby

The drugs most commonly used illicitly fall broadly into three main categories: sedative or depressant (opiates, opioids, benzodiazepines, cannabis), stimulant (amphetamines, cocaine) and perception-altering or hallucinogenic (LSD, high-dose cannabis).

Drug misuse is illegal and self-reporting of drug use is often unreliable. In addition patterns and levels of use are not constant and polydrug use is common even in the presence of prescribed substitute medication. Many reported data derive from relatively small samples, so for all these reasons reliable data on effects of drug use on pregnancy outcome are difficult to obtain.

There have been inconsistent reports of increased congenital abnormalities, but no good evidence of significant teratogenesis from the drugs most commonly used illicitly. For example, while there are conflicting data on an association between cleft palate and benzodiazepine use, with the balance in favour of an increased risk, the absolute risk remains low. Similarly underdevelopment of organs or limbs due to the vasoconstrictor effect of cocaine is rarely seen. Fetal alcohol syndrome appears to have varying genetic susceptibility and consequently varying prevalence, but the full syndrome including craniofacial abnormalities is uncommon in the UK. In all these situations any possible increase in fetal abnormalities is not clinically important and is not the most important issue for those with problem drug use. Significant misuse of drugs in pregnancy is associated with higher rates of perinatal mortality and morbidity, but this is only partly due to the effect of the drugs, with a major contribution from socioeconomic deprivation and other social problems that either predispose to drug use or are a consequence of drug use. Low birth weight is the most frequently observed adverse outcome due to reduced fetal growth and/or preterm delivery, while increased rates of sudden infant death are reported. These outcomes are all increased in the presence of socioeconomic deprivation and associated factors such as cigarette smoking. Neonatal withdrawal symptoms due to opiate/opioid and/or benzodiazepine use often pose the biggest management challenge as well as causing considerable maternal distress (Table 12.1).

Sedative drugs

Opiates/opioids

Heroin: Opiates and opioids are the most commonly misused drugs, of which heroin is the most frequently reported by those seeking help for addiction problems. Heroin obtained illicitly is in a brown powder containing various other substances that can themselves be harmful. It is commonly smoked in cigarette form or heated over tin foil and inhaled (chasing the dragon) or injected. There is no evidence of teratogenesis, but heroin causes reduced fetal growth [11]. Its use in pregnancy is associated with increased perinatal mortality and morbidity, attributable largely to increased rates of low birth weight due to intrauterine growth retardation with or without preterm delivery [12,13]. An increased risk of sudden infant death syndrome (SIDS) is also reported [14] and thought to

Table 12.1 Characteristics of commonly abused drugs

Drug	Action	Effects	Substitution	Neonatal withdrawal symptoms	Breastfeeding
Opiates/Opioids					
Heroin	Sedative	Increased IUGR, Preterm labour, SIDS	Yes	Yes	Yes, if stable (successful establishment evidence of adequate stability)
Methadone	Sedative	Increased IUGR, SIDS	N/A	Yes	Yes
Buprenorphine	Sedative	As heroin probably	Yes	Yes	Yes
Dihydrocodeine	Sedative	As heroin	Yes	Yes	Yes, as heroin
Benzodiazepines	Sedative	Increased cleft palate	Short term to cover withdrawal only	Yes	Yes, as heroin
Amphetamines	Stimulant	None significant	No	No	Yes, as heroin
Ecstasy	Stimulant	None	No	No	Yes
Cocaine	Stimulant	Increased placental abruption, PROM, SIDS Possible increase in IUGR Preterm labour	No	No	Yes, as heroin
LSD	Hallucinogenic	None	No	No	Yes
Cannabis	Sedative (hallucinogenic in high dose)	None	No	No	Yes

IUGR, intrauterine growth retardation; PROM, premature rupture of membranes; SIDS, sudden infant death syndrome.

be related to the observation of reduced fetal breathing and reduced fetal response to carbon dioxide [15]. Heroin has a relatively short half-life, so many of the adverse effects are caused or exaggerated by repeated minor degrees of withdrawal. Withdrawal causes smooth muscle spasm; uterine contractions may precipitate preterm delivery or abortion (although the latter is difficult to quantify) while placental vasoconstriction may cause fetal compromise and reduced intrauterine growth. Spasm of the fetal gut may lead to antepartum passage of meconium. Acute maternal withdrawal of opiates has been reported to be associated with increased levels of amniotic fluid catecholamines [16]. For this reason it has been widely held that antenatal detoxification is dangerous and should only be undertaken in mid-trimester if at all and then only at very slow rates. However, experience in Glasgow has demonstrated that in practice, despite the theoretical risks, detoxification at any speed and at any stage of pregnancy is not unacceptably hazardous to the fetus [17]. However, the same cannot be said of reversal with naloxone, which may precipitate severe antepartum fetal distress or shock in the neonate and should be used only with extreme caution. Since prescribed opiate substitutes do not carry the same risk of preterm labour as heroin, pregnant women using heroin should always be stabilised on substitute opiate medication without delay. Stability during pregnancy is more important than abstinence, and subsequent detoxification should only be undertaken if it is the woman's choice and the timing is appropriate with a reasonable prospect of success. However, pregnancy is rarely a good time for women to attempt detoxification and since stability can be affected by various factors and life events, in practice the dose of substitute medication should be increased or decreased accordingly with the aim of maintenance at the lowest dose compatible with reasonable stability. Methadone remains the substitute of choice but buprenorphine, previously extensively misused in Scotland, is now prescribed as an opiate substitute, more often in a reducing than a maintenance regime. However, as a maintenance therapy it has no benefits compared to methadone, so there is no indication to switch from one drug to the other during pregnancy. Other substitute drugs are available but are either unevaluated or contraindicated in pregnancy.

Heroin causes withdrawal symptoms in the neonate, with timing of onset and severity depending on pattern and level of maternal use. If used up to the time of delivery, symptoms usually appear within 24 hours, increasing over the next day or two and resolving within a week. The severity of symptoms is largely dose dependent but can be increased by intrapartum fetal asphyxia or other causes of morbidity and decreased by prematurity with immaturity of the neurological system. Other opiates/opioids such as dihydrocodeine, which is frequently misused, and benzodiazepines, prescribed or illicit, also cause neonatal withdrawal and so unexpectedly severe or prolonged symptoms may reflect polydrug use. Maternal dosage therefore cannot be used accurately to predict the likelihood or severity of withdrawal; nor can the baby's condition be taken to accurately reflect the mother's level of use.

Heroin is present in breast milk, but this means that breastfeeding can be helpful in avoiding or minimising withdrawal symptoms in the baby. It should be pointed out that women using heroin should be stabilised on prescribed substitute medication during pregnancy, so the question of breastfeeding by women using heroin should rarely arise. Nevertheless in the absence of contraindications, breastfeeding by women using heroin should be advocated, provided drug use is reasonably stable. Women whose drug use is very heavy or chaotic are rarely able to breastfeed successfully either because of inadequate milk production or because of intoxication or lack of application, and successful establishment of breastfeeding is therefore in itself an indicator of adequate stability. Breastfeeding should not be suddenly discontinued, since this might precipitate withdrawal symptoms in the baby. Few women who have successfully established breastfeeding will stop suddenly but it is important that they are aware of the risks of so doing. Breastfeeding increases the risk of vertical transmission of HIV and so maternal HIV infection is a contraindication to breastfeeding. There is no evidence that HCV infection is transmitted by breastfeeding and indeed available evidence suggests this is not the case; therefore, breastfeeding is not contraindicated for women who are HCV PCR positive. All babies born to socially disadvantaged mothers and especially babies born to drug-using mothers are extremely vulnerable with most to gain from breastfeeding. The greater the level of maternal drug use, the greater the risks of neonatal withdrawal symptoms, low birthweight and cot death and consequently the greater the potential benefits of breastfeeding. In the absence of maternal HIV infection, all drug-using women, regardless of drugs used or level or pattern of use, should therefore be encouraged to breastfeed. It must be recognised, however, that breastfeeding is not widely acceptable among disadvantaged women and may be completely unacceptable to many including those with a history of childhood sexual abuse. While strong encouragement is required to help many drug-using women overcome their disinclination, it is important to recognise those who are unable to breastfeed and help them to accept the decision to bottle-feed without undue feelings of guilt.

Information about long-term effects of drug use on child development is difficult to obtain because of difficulties in maintaining contact and difficult to interpret because of confounding factors. It has been reported that maternal heroin use in pregnancy is associated with ongoing growth impairment and behavioural disturbances [18], but genetic, antenatal, and postnatal environmental factors may also be significant. Long-term outcome is reported to be better among women maintained on methadone [19], but this may reflect that compared to women using heroin women on methadone usually have greater stability of drug use as well as other aspects of lifestyle with more regular attendance for antenatal care.

Methadone: Methadone is an opioid available as tablet, linctus or injectable liquid and is the most commonly prescribed substitution drug for those dependent on opiates and opioids. It is socially beneficial because it removes the need to finance drug use by crime, stabilises lifestyle and brings users into contact with support services. Medically it is preferable to heroin because, in addition to being legal, it is pure, is usually prescribed in the oral linctus form and, of particular benefit in pregnancy, it has a long half-life with a duration of action in excess of 24 hours. This eliminates the fluctuations in blood levels of drug that occur with heroin use and which are harmful to the fetus and in particular – as previously stated – methadone protects the fetus from the increased risk of preterm labour associated with heroin use. Again as in the case of heroin use, antenatal maternal detoxification from methadone is acceptably safe at any speed and at any stage of pregnancy. Whether or at what rate the dose of methadone is reduced should be individually agreed and dictated by the woman's wishes and her ability to cope. As already noted, it may at times be necessary to increase rather than decrease the dose, and throughout pregnancy the appropriate dose is the lowest that is compatible with reasonable stability. It should be remembered that methadone as an opioid shares many effects with the drug(s) it replaces, and as the dose increases the cost/benefit balance will shift. Methadone is associated with reduced birth weight [19], which becomes more significant as the dose increases. Like heroin it is reported to increase the risk of SIDS [20] and reduced fetal breathing and response to carbon dioxide are observed [15]. It is often advised that it is necessary to increase the dose of methadone in late pregnancy, but in practice this is not the case and indeed women often achieve their most significant reductions in dosage, as impending delivery with the prospect of neonatal withdrawal symptoms strengthens their motivation. At this stage it is important to ensure that their goals are realistic and to emphasise the importance of stability rather than abstinence. It is also important to remember that such reductions achieved in the short term may not be sustainable in the long term, and it may be necessary to increase the methadone dose postnatally to ensure ongoing stability. Objectives in substitute prescribing may therefore be rather different in pregnancy.

In the past some have argued that substitution therapy with methadone is not justified for non-injecting use of heroin or for illicit use of other opiates/opioids such as dihydrocodeine. However, prescription of methadone removes the cost of illicit drug use and consequently the need to engage in illegal activities, stabilises lifestyle and brings women into contact with services, and together with the fetal benefits from methadone's longer half-life justifies prescription of substitute opiate/opioid medication for all women using illicit opiates/opioids. While there are no good data on use of dihydrocodeine in pregnancy, anecdotally it is associated with higher neonatal morbidity than methadone, justifying transfer of pregnant women from prescribed dihydrocodeine to methadone. While the greatest increase in perinatal mortality is reported to occur with continued use of heroin on top of prescribed methadone, this refers to significant use of both drugs and is probably attributable to instability of lifestyle and associated factors [21] rather than direct effects of the drugs per se; unlimited increases in methadone dosage in (sometimes futile) pursuit of total abstinence from all illicit drugs may therefore be less beneficial to the fetus than very occasional use of non-injected heroin on top of a more modest dose of methadone when this is associated with stability of lifestyle. In pregnancy there may therefore be a lower threshold for prescribing methadone, but a more conservative approach to dosage.

Methadone also causes withdrawal symptoms in the neonate but because of the longer half-life, these occur later than with heroin. They are often apparent within 48 hours and are usually obvious by 3–5 days of age, resolving within 10 days or so but occasionally lasting longer. Overall, the severity of neonatal withdrawal symptoms is partly dose dependent, but also influenced by the speed of metabolism of methadone (which has a genetic component) and modified by other perinatal factors. Unexpectedly severe or prolonged symptoms may be a consequence of polydrug use, especially when this involves benzodiazepine use.

Methadone is also present in breast milk and the arguments already given in favour of breastfeeding by women using opiates/opioids apply here. For women stable on long-term maintenance methadone, the question of how long to continue breastfeeding is often raised. While prolonged breastfeeding especially in the presence of a high dose of methadone might not be desirable, there is no obvious end point and decisions should be individually made; however, for all women on methadone, it would be reasonable to continue for at least 6 months or so to achieve maximum benefits for the baby.

The problems of assessing long-term effects of methadone use on child development are similar to those for use of heroin. However, it seems likely from the limited data available that maternal methadone therapy per se is not detrimental [19] and adverse environmental factors are probably of greater significance [22].

Buprenorphine: This is a partial opiate agonist available as sublingual tablet or injectable liquid. It is marketed as a mild/moderate analgesic but, contrary to initial claims, has addictive properties and is therefore misused. The sublingual tablets are highly soluble and therefore injectable. In Scotland in the 1980s buprenorphine was extensively misused at doses many times in the recommended therapeutic range and was the foremost drug of choice among those addicted to opiates/opioids. At dosages associated with misuse, it has effects similar to those of heroin with increased rates of low birth weight due to growth retardation and/or preterm delivery. Buprenorphine is now used as substitute medication, especially in detoxification on the grounds that it is claimed to be easier to withdraw than methadone. Trials of use of buprenorphine are ongoing but the volume of data on its use in pregnancy is still much smaller than that on use of methadone in pregnancy. It has been claimed that buprenorphine causes less severe neonatal withdrawals than methadone, but in practice there seems little difference. The severity of neonatal withdrawal symptoms is influenced by many other factors that affect neonatal morbidity and so comparison can be difficult. However, data relating to its illicit use in pregnancy by several hundred women in Glasgow, while uncontrolled, suggest that outcomes were comparable to those with methadone but while the amounts used illicitly were many times greater than recommended therapeutic doses, they were still much lower than those recommended for treatment of drug misuse. There is therefore no indication to change substitute medication during pregnancy from methadone to buprenorphine or vice versa.

Buprenorphine also causes neonatal withdrawal symptoms, which are similar in timing to those due to heroin. Again buprenorphine is present in breast milk and in the absence of contraindications, breastfeeding should be advocated.

Dihydrocodeine: Marketed as an analgesic for moderate pain, dihydrocodeine is available in oral and injectable forms. The latter is a controlled drug but the oral form is not and is consequently sometimes prescribed as opiate/opioid substitution by doctors reluctant to prescribe methadone. There are insufficient data on its use in pregnancy at doses associated with prescribed substitution or with misuse to allow comparison with use of methadone or heroin in pregnancy. In particular it is not clear whether it increases the risk of preterm labour. However, anecdotally it is observed to be associated with reduced birth weight and with more frequent meconium staining of the liquor, and while theoretically these effects could be related to dihydrocodeine's short duration of action, they are also observed with the slow release preparations.

Dihydrocodeine causes neonatal withdrawal symptoms that are usually apparent within 24 hours. Again anecdotally these symptoms may be severe and prolonged and apparently out of proportion with the level of drug use. Some women top up their prescribed substitution therapy with oral dihydrocodeine in the belief that the latter does not constitute 'drug use' and as in the case of topping up with other illicit drugs, but more marked than when topping up with other opiates/opioids, this may be a factor when methadone withdrawals seem unexpectedly severe or prolonged. While these observations are purely anecdotal, controlled scientific data are difficult to obtain and these effects are observed with sufficient frequency to justify advising against use of dihydrocodeine in pregnancy.

Dihydrocodeine is present in breast milk. During pregnancy and after delivery, efforts should be directed towards cessation of use or substitution by another less harmful drug such as methadone. Nevertheless the overall benefits of breastfeeding for these vulnerable babies are such that breastfeeding should be encouraged regardless of whether these efforts are successful.

Other opiates/opioids: A variety of other drugs are misused, including morphine (various preparations), dipipanone (Diconal), pethidine, dextromoramide (Palfium), pentazocine (Fortral), dextropropoxyphene (with paracetamol as Distalgesic or co-proxamol) and various codeine-containing analgesics. In general they have symptoms similar to those described for the more common opiates/opioids although there may be both quantitative and qualitative differences. Many of the analgesics prescribed for mild/moderate pain will therefore adversely affect the fetus if used alone and will also contribute to and exacerbate neonatal withdrawal symptoms if used in combination with other opiates/opioids. The possibility of misuse should always be borne in mind when prescribing such analgesics especially if requested on a recurrent basis and their potentially harmful effects on the fetus should be remembered when prescribing to women who may become pregnant. A full history of all drug use, prescribed, over the counter and illicit should be taken from all pregnant women at the booking visit and women should be told to notify staff of any subsequent use during the pregnancy. If this is omitted, however, the unexpected development in a baby of symptoms suggestive of drug withdrawal should prompt the belated taking of a drug history.

Benzodiazepines

Legal prescription of benzodiazepines peaked around 1980 but as this has diminished, illicit use of a wide range of preparations has increased particularly among young people. They are used illicitly both orally and by injection with temazepam particularly liable to be injected. As already discussed, benzodiazepine use in combination with other drugs especially opiates/opioids is common and the practice of injecting temazepam together with heroin was a major problem in Scotland [6]. Illicit use of temazepam has, however, been largely replaced by that of diazepam with a reduction in injecting use of benzodiazepines, reflecting an overall reduction in injecting as already noted. Benzodiazepines are used in association with cocaine to reduce the depressant effects that follow its use and together with opiates/opioids to increase the pleasurable effects. The doses of benzodiazepines used illicitly are often very high and compared to women who use opiates/opioids alone, women who also use benzodiazepines are in all respects very unstable [3].

There has been considerable debate over whether the incidence of cleft palate is increased in association with benzodiazepine use. While current evidence does indicate an increased relative risk, the absolute risk remains low and is of limited clinical significance [23]. Similarly, reported associations with pyloric stenosis, cardiac defects, inguinal hernias and craniofacial defects [24,25], if they exist, are not clinically significant; in Glasgow among several hundred women who used benzodiazepines at all stages of pregnancy, often in association with opiates/opioids, often by injection and in more than 90% of cases in combination with smoking, no increased rate of anomalies has been observed (Hepburn M., unpublished data). Growth retardation as reported in one small study [26] has been observed but in the presence of variable polydrug use and instability of lifestyle, the precise contribution from benzodiazepine use per se is difficult to quantify. Benzodiazepines cause withdrawal symptoms in the baby that, especially with shorter acting drugs such as temazepam, are often evident in the first 24–48 hours and can be very troublesome and often prolonged. They are often very similar to those caused by opiates/opioids and where the drugs are used in combination, it may be difficult to distinguish effects from each type and the net effect is of severe and prolonged withdrawals. This effect is often heightened by the adverse effects of benzodiazepine use on the mothers' parenting skills.

There is no evidence that substitution therapy reduces the level of use or improves stability of drug use or lifestyle, so management should be directed towards maternal withdrawal. If sudden, this may precipitate convulsions in the mother. However, regardless of level of use complete withdrawal can be safely achieved within a week using a longer acting drug such as diazepam (which is also an effective anticonvulsant) with an initial level as low as 30–40 mg/day in divided doses and daily reduction of one dose in rotation. There should be no attempt to reduce levels of opiate/opioid use during withdrawal from benzodiazepines and indeed it may be helpful to increase the dose of methadone or other opiate substitute until the woman is stable off benzodiazepines. Relapse is not uncommon and repeated attempts at benzodiazepine withdrawal may be necessary. This is not an indication that it should not have been attempted in the first place, since any reduction in use even if not sustained in the long term will be of benefit to the fetus. It is also important to remember that subsequent over-enthusiastic or unrealistic reduction in methadone dosage may precipitate resumption of top up use of benzodiazepines.

The benzodiazepines that are commonly used illicitly pass into the breast milk. With low levels of use the advantages of breastfeeding will outweigh any possible disadvantages; at higher levels of maternal use successful establishment of breastfeeding is unlikely as in the case of maternal opiate/opioid use. It is therefore reasonable to encourage all women using benzodiazepines to attempt breastfeeding.

Stimulants

Amphetamines

Amphetamine (α-methylphenethylamine) can be swallowed, snorted, smoked or injected. Illicitly obtained amphetamine is highly impure, with only a small amount of amphetamine mixed with a variety of other substances some of which may have harmful effects. There are no specific effects associated with amphetamine use in pregnancy and with intermittent or recreational use no evidence of effect on pregnancy outcome. With high continuous levels of use, growth retardation may occur but unstable lifestyle with poor nutrition will be contributory factors. In high dosage and especially by injection amphetamine use is more harmful; for example, consequences reported by the Edinburgh Poisons Bureau include bleeding disorders and abdominal pain, a combination that may suggest placental abruption. Such a presentation is, however, very rare. At common levels of use, short-term increases in pulse and blood pressure have little effect but in all cases the clinical picture may be confused by effects of substances used to cut the amphetamines or by drugs used in combination with it.

There is debate about the role of substitution therapy for amphetamine users. Its use is sometimes justified for heavy and/or injecting users on the grounds that it may bring them into contact with support services and reduce levels of injecting. However, there is no evidence that substitution therapy is beneficial in the management of pregnant amphetamine users. Amphetamines do not cause withdrawal symptoms in the baby and breastfeeding, in the absence of specific contraindications, should be encouraged.

Ecstasy

Ecstasy use is largely recreational; it does not lead to significant physical dependence and even at high levels is not usually associated with the instability of lifestyle and consequent problems seen with use of opiates/opioids or benzodiazepines. There is no evidence of adverse effects on pregnancy nor of withdrawal symptoms in the baby, and breastfeeding is not contraindicated.

Cocaine

Cocaine is available as cocaine hydrochloride and as crack cocaine, the latter produced by heating cocaine hydrochloride with sodium bicarbonate. Cocaine hydrochloride illicitly obtained is impure and the powder is either sniffed/snorted or injected and is sometimes injected in combination with heroin (speedball). Crack cocaine is pure crystalline cocaine which is usually smoked but can be injected if first made soluble by mixing with an acid such as vitamin C. Use of cocaine by snorting is commonly recreational but injected cocaine and crack cocaine by any route are associated with dependent use, and polydrug use is common. There is no suitable or effective substitution therapy for cocaine, so many users do not present to services but increasingly, pregnant women with drug problems may report use of cocaine along with other drugs.

The difficulties in identifying and quantifying specific drug effects on pregnancy outcome and factors that influence reporting have been well illustrated in the case of cocaine. Cocaine is widely regarded as a particularly harmful drug if used in pregnancy. There are numerous reports of adverse outcomes including congenital malformations [26], spontaneous abortion [27], placental abruption [27,28], growth retardation [29,30], preterm delivery [29,31] and SIDS [32]. Cocaine is a powerful vasoconstrictor and vascular compromise has been suggested as a common aetiology for many fetal abnormalities including limb reduction defects and non-duodenal intestinal atresia, symmetrical growth retardation, spontaneous abortion and placental abruption [33]. Such findings are inconsistent with other reports of no increase in congenital malformations or preterm delivery [30]. It is widely acknowledged that the nature and/or extent of adverse outcomes is difficult to determine due to the frequent presence of other factors such as low socioeconomic status and associated problems. However, there is good evidence of a bias against publication of studies that do not report adverse outcomes [34]. There is no doubt that heavy uncontrolled use of cocaine together with an unstable and unhealthy lifestyle will increase the risk of adverse pregnancy outcomes; it seems likely that lesser recreational use does not have similar effects.

Cocaine does not cause neonatal withdrawal symptoms. Problems in the baby, if they occur, are attributable to antenatal complications. Breastfeeding is not invariably contraindicated in the presence of any cocaine use; decisions about breastfeeding should be made individually on the basis of presence or absence of contraindications and stability of lifestyle.

Hallucinogenic drugs

LSD

Use of LSD in pregnancy is usually intermittent and recreational. No specific problems have been demonstrated in association with its use in pregnancy and it does not cause withdrawal symptoms in the neonate. Substitution therapy is neither available nor necessary.

Cannabis

Cannabis use is widespread in the UK and therefore relatively common among pregnant women. It can be taken orally but is usually smoked either on its own or together with tobacco. The individual contributions of cannabis and tobacco to observed outcomes are difficult to determine, but it has been reported to cause no increase in congenital malformations, early pregnancy loss or obstetric complications [35]. Nevertheless uncertainty remains and concomitant tobacco use is harmful and so any advice should be to reduce levels of use as much as possible during pregnancy.

Conclusion

While abstinence may be best for the fetus, it is frequently an unrealistic objective. Judgmental attitudes by health-care professionals are inappropriate and unhelpful, and drug-using women should be given balanced information which is not unduly alarmist. In view of their potentially high-risk pregnancies their care should be medically led but much of it can be delivered by midwives in the community. Management should address social as well as medical problems and should be provided by a multidisciplinary team in line with national guidelines [36].

Key points

- Amenorrhoea is common among heroin users but conception can still occur
- Naloxone can precipitate severe antepartum fetal distress in heroin users
- Breastfeeding can minimise neonatal withdrawal in heroin and/or benzodiazepine users
- All drug-using women should be encouraged to breastfeed unless they are known to be HIV positive

References

1 Home Office. Statistics of drug addicts notified to the Home Office, United Kingdom, 1994. Home Office Statistical Bulletin 17/95. London: HMSO; 1995.

2 Department of Health. Drug misuse statistics. Department of Health Statistical Bulletin 1996/24. London: Department of Health; 1996.

3 Darke S. The Use of benzodiazepines amongst injecting drug users. *Drug Alcohol Rev* 1995;**13**:63–9.

4 Seivewright N, Donmall M, Daly C. Benzodiazepines in the illicit drugs scene: the UK picture and some dilemmas. *Int J Drug Policy* 1993;**4**(1):42–8.

5 Information Services Division. Drug Misuse Statistics Scotland. Edinburgh: Common Services Agency; 1999.

6 Forsyth AJM, Farquhar D, Gemmell M, Shewan D, Davies JB. The dual use of opioids and temazepam by drug injectors in Glasgow (Scotland). *Drug Alcohol Depend* May 1993;**32**(3):277–80.

7 Information Services Division. Drug Misuse Statistics Scotland. Edinburgh: Common Services Agency; 2005.

8 Rementeria JL, Janakammal S, Hollander M. Multiple births in drug addicted women. *Am J Obstet Gynecol* 1975;**122**:958–60.

9 Bai J, Greenwald E, Caterini H, Kaminetzky H. Drug related menstrual aberrations. *Obstet Gynecol* 1974;**44**:713–9.

10 Perlmutter J. Heroin addiction and pregnancy. *Obstet Gynecol Surv* 1974;**29**:439–46.

11 Naeye RL, Blanc W, Leblanc W, Khatamee MA. Fetal complications of maternal heroin addiction: abnormal growth infections and episodes of stress. *J Pediatr* December 1973;**83**(6):1055–61.

12 Kandall SR, Albin S, Lowinson J, Berle B, Eidelman AI, Gartner LM. Differential effects of maternal heroin and methadone use on birth weight. *Pediatrics* November 1976;**58**(5):681–5.

13 Zelson C, Rubio E, Wasserman E. Neonatal narcotic addiction: 10 year observation. *Pediatrics* August 1971;**48**(2):178–89.

14 Kandall SR, Gaines JJ. Maternal substance use and subsequent sudden infant death syndrome (SIDS) in offspring. *Neurotoxicol Teratol* 1991;**13**:235–40.

15 Ward SLD, Schuetz S, Krishna V, et al. Abnormal sleeping ventilatory pattern in infants of substance-abusing mothers. *Am J Dis Child* 1986;**140**:1015–20.

16 Zuspan FP, Gumpel JA, Mejia-Zelaya A, Davis R. Fetal stress from methadone withdrawal. *Am J Obstet Gynecol* 1975;**122**:43–6.

17 Hepburn M. Drugs of abuse. In: Cockburn F (ed.), *Advances in Perinatal Medicine*. London: Parthenon Publishing; 1997:120–4.

18 Wilson GS, Desmond MM, Verniaud WM. Early development of infants of heroin addicted mothers. *Am J Dis Child* 1973;**126**(4):457–62.

19 Blinick G, Jerez E, Wallach RC. Methadone maintenance, pregnancy, and progeny. *JAMA* 1973;**225**(5):477–9.

20 Pierson PS, Howard P, Kleber HD. Sudden death in infants born to methadone-maintained addicts. *JAMA* 1972;**220**:1733–4.

21 Hulse GK, Milne DR, English CD, Holman CDJ. Assessing the relationship between maternal opiate use and neonatal mortality. *Addiction* 1998;**93**(7):1033–42.

22 Strauss ME, Lessen-Firestone JK, Starr RH, Jr, Ostrea EM. Behavior of narcotics addicted newborns. *Child Dev* December 1975;**46**(4):887–93.

23 Dolovich LR, Addis A, Vaillancourt J, Power J, Koren G, Einarson T. Benzodiazepine use in pregnancy and major malformations or oral cleft: meta-analysis of cohort and case-control studies. *BMJ* 1998;**317**:839–43.

24 Bracken MB, Holford TR. Exposure to prescribed drugs in pregnancy and association with congenital malformations. *Obstet Gynecol* 1981;**58**:336–44.

25 Laegreid L, Olegard R, Walstrom J, Conradi N. Teratogenic effects of benzodiazepine use during pregnancy. *J Paediatr* 1989;**114**:123–31.

26 Bingol N, Fuchs M, Diaz V, Stone RK, Gromisch DS. Teratogenicity of cocaine in humans. *J Pediatr* 1987;**110**:93–6.

27 Chasnoff IJ, Burns WJ, Schnoll SH, Burns KA. Cocaine use in pregnancy. *N Engl J Med* 1985;**313**:666–9.

28 Acker D, Sachs BP, Tracey KJ, Wise WE. Abruptio placentae associated with cocaine use. *Am J Obstet Gynecol* 1983;**146**:220–1.

29 Chouteau M, Brickner Namerow P, Leppert P. The effect of cocaine abuse on birth weight and gestational age. *Obstet Gynecol* 1988;**72**: 351–4.

30 Zuckerman B, Frank DA, Hingson R, et al. Effect of maternal marijuana and cocaine use on fetal growth. *N Engl J Med* 1989;**320**:762–8.

31 Oro AS, Dixon SD. Perinatal cocaine and methamphetamine exposure: maternal and neonatal correlates. *J Pediatr* 1987;**111**:571–8.

32 Chasnoff IJ, Burns KA, Burns WJ. Cocaine use in pregnancy: perinatal morbidity and mortality. *Neurotoxicol Teratol* 1987;**9**:291–3.

33 Hoyme HE, Jones KL, Dixon SD, et al. Prenatal cocaine exposure and fetal vascular disruption. *Pediatrics* 1990;**85**:743–7.

34 Koren G, Graham K, Shear H, Einarson T. Bias against the null hypothesis: the reproductive hazards of cocaine. *Lancet* 1989;**2**:1440–2.

35 Fried P. Marijuana and human pregnancy. In: Chasnoff IJ (ed.), *Drug Use in Pregnancy: Mother and Child*. Norwell, MA: MTP Press; 1986:64–74.

36 Local Government Drugs Forum (LGDF). Drug using parents: policy guidelines for inter-agency working. In: *Standing Conference on Drug Abuse (SCODA)*. London: LGA; 1997.

CHAPTER 13

Prescribing for the pregnant traveller

Pauline A. Hurley

Prescriptions, which need to be considered for the pregnant traveller, are immunisations prior to travel, drugs that may be taken for travel sickness, malaria prophylaxis and the treatment of traveller's diarrhoea. This article aims to give an overview of the above and suggestions for the pregnant traveller's 'first-aid kit'.

Immunisations

No vaccine, toxoid or immunoglobulin can be regarded as entirely safe in pregnancy. Acute illness, either as a result of giving a vaccine [1,2] or as a result of contracting an infection, brings with it the risk of premature labour, with consequent morbidity and mortality or the risk of in utero infection. Immunisation should be given in pregnancy only if there is a clearly defined risk and travel to endemic areas cannot be avoided. In general, live vaccines should be avoided in pregnancy, including BCG, MMR, yellow fever and oral preparations for polio.

Table 13.1 summarises the guidelines for immunisation in pregnancy and Table 13.2 provides the current recommendations for travel derived from the *British National Formulary* [3] and the American College of Obstetricians and Gynaecologist Committee Opinion paper No. 282 [4].

It should be noted that the World Health Organisation no longer recommends cholera vaccination for international travellers and it should no longer be an entry requirement into any foreign country

Prescribing in Pregnancy, 4th edition. Edited by Peter Rubin and Margaret Ramsay,
 ISBN: 978-1-4051-4712-5.

Table 13.1 Guidelines for immunisation in pregnancy

Possibility of harm in pregnancy remote			
None			
There would appear to be no adverse effects outside the first trimester: animal studies have not demonstrated a fetal risk but no controlled studies in women			
Hepatitis A	Immune globulin	Hepatitis B	Immune globulin
Rabies	Immune globulin	Tetanus	Immune globulin
Varicella zoster	Immune globulin		
Should only be given if there is a proper indication and risk of infection: animal studies have not demonstrated an adverse effect but there are no studies in women			
BCG	Vaccine	Cholera	Vaccine
Diphtheria	Toxoid	*E. Coli*	Vaccine
Influenza	Vaccine	Meningitis	Vaccine
Plague	Vaccine	*Pneumococcus*	Vaccine
Polio	Vaccine	Tetanus	Toxoid
Tularaemia	Vaccine	Typhoid	Vaccine
The benefits of vaccination may be acceptable: there is positive evidence of fetal risk			
Yellow fever	Vaccine		
The vaccine is contraindicated in pregnancy			
Measles	Vaccine		
Mumps	Vaccine		
Rubella	Vaccine		
Smallpox	Vaccine		
Varicella	Vaccine		

[5]. The vaccine is not effective in that it only provides limited personal protection and does not prevent the spread of this water-borne acute diarrhoeal disease.

Diphtheria

Widespread immunisation against diphtheria in childhood has virtually eliminated this disease from the UK but diphtheria toxoid is recommended if neither booster nor immunisation has been given in the previous 10 years and travel to a high-risk area (Africa or the Indian subcontinent) cannot be avoided. Diphtheria and tetanus boosters are now commonly given in combination [3,4].

Table 13.2 Current recommendations for immunisation and travel

Area of the world	Recommended for all areas	Recommended for some areas
Indian subcontinent	Hepatitis A Polio Tetanus Typhoid TB	Yellow fever Meningococcal meningitis
Far East	Hepatitis A Tetanus Polio TB	Japanese encephalitis
Middle East	Hepatitis A Tetanus Polio TB	Meningococcal meningitis
Africa	Hepatitis A Typhoid Tetanus TB	Yellow fever Meningococcal meningitis Polio
Central and South America	Hepatitis A TB Typhoid Tetanus Polio	Yellow fever
Eastern Europe	Hepatitis A Polio Tetanus	
Areas out of immediate medical attention or rural stays >30 days	Rabies Hepatitis B	

Tetanus

Tetanus contracted during pregnancy is associated with high morbidity, with neonatal tetanus mortality being in the region of 65% [6]. There appear to be no adverse effects from giving toxoid in pregnancy and the American College of Obstetricians and Gynaecologists endorses its use in pregnancy, particularly if the woman may deliver in unhygienic circumstances [7]. A booster is recommended every 10 years. A total of five doses are said to convey lifelong protection, but a booster is recommended in the event of any tetanus-prone injury.

Meningococcal meningitis

At present there is no effective vaccine against the B serogroup of the meningococcus, which is the commonest cause of meningitis in the UK. A vaccine is available as a purified bacterial capsular polysaccharide mix of serogroups A and C, W135 and Y, but this is only recommended if there is a true risk of infection. This would apply to those travelling to sub-Saharan Africa, Delhi, Nepal, Bhutan, Pakistan and Haj pilgrims travelling to Saudi Arabia. Vaccination conveys protection for 3–5 years [3].

Typhoid

There are three vaccines available for the prevention of typhoid: a monovalent whole cell vaccine which is heat killed and phenol preserved, a typhoid Vi polysaccharide antigen containing Vi antigen from the bacterial capsule and an oral live attenuated vaccine. The live oral vaccine is contraindicated in pregnancy. No data are available on the safety of the other vaccines in pregnancy and none are 100% effective and certainly do not provide a substitute for careful hygiene and food preparation. Vaccination conveys protection for 3 years. Vi capsular polysaccharide vaccine is often given in combination with hepatitis A vaccine [3].

Hepatitis A

The risk of acquiring hepatitis A is no different for the pregnant woman than any other traveller. Whilst it is usually associated with travel to rural areas in developing countries, it has been reported in tourists travelling to destinations closer to home. Whilst maternal infection is said not to be associated with perinatal transmission, placental abruption and premature delivery of an infected infant has been reported [8].

A hepatitis A vaccine is available for active immunisation, but there are no data available on its safety in pregnancy. Ten-year protection is achieved by giving three doses over 6 months. An accelerated course can be given to travellers. Theoretically, as it is not a live vaccine the risk is small but there are concerns regarding its use in pregnancy, as a febrile response to vaccination is not uncommon.

Passive immunisation with human normal immunoglobulin is the usual mode of conveying protection for the traveller, if they have not previously received hepatitis A vaccination. It gives up to 4 months' protection and carries no apparent risks in pregnancy [7].

Hepatitis B

Hepatitis B infection in pregnancy can cause severe disease in the mother and chronic infection in the neonate [9]. All pregnant women in the UK are screened at the beginning of pregnancy and if they are found to be negative by serology for past infection or immunisation, they can be given recombinant hepatitis B vaccine in the unlikely event that they will be travelling to endemic areas and risk exposure to blood or blood products [4].

Yellow fever

Yellow fever is spread by the infected mosquito, but confined to tropical Africa and South America. During epidemics fatality for unimmunised adults can exceed 50%. The vaccine is a live attenuated freeze-dried vaccine. The risks to the fetus are unknown, and it should be regarded as contraindicated in pregnancy. There may be circumstances, however, when the risks of the disease outweigh the risk of immunisation. Travel to areas requiring documentary evidence of immunisation should therefore be avoided in pregnancy [1].

The areas of greatest risk of exposure to the above are the Far and Middle East, Central and South America, Asia, Eastern Europe and endemic areas of Africa. Travel to these areas is best avoided in pregnancy.

Polio

Immunisation against polio is recommended for most areas of travel. Oral live vaccine (Sabin) is no longer recommended, except during outbreaks, and is contraindicated in pregnancy, although no fetal damage has been reported following inadvertent administration during pregnancy. Injectable killed vaccine (Salk) can be used and conveys protection for 10 years. For travellers it is commonly given in combination with diphtheria and tetanus [3].

Rabies

Immunisation against rabies in pregnancy is recommended only if there is a significant risk and there is no rapid access to a medical facility, which can provide post-exposure prophylaxis. A full course of three doses is required to confer 3–5-year protection [3].

Malaria prophylaxis

It should be remembered that no drug regimen ensures complete protection against malaria. Complications of the disease are more severe in pregnancy, and mid-trimester abortion, preterm delivery and low birth weight are direct complications [7]. Transplacental transmission can occur with devastating consequences for the neonate. Dehydration, thrombocytopenia, splenic rupture and seizures have all been reported. There is also evidence that placental malarial infection may increase the risk of transmission of other bloodborne pathogens such as HIV [10].

Avoidance of mosquito bites by physical means is the best advice. This will include wearing protective clothing, trousers and long-sleeved shirts together with the use of insect repellents. Many preparations contain DEET (14C-*N*,*N*-diethyl-*m*-tolumide), which has been shown to be absorbed through the skin and to cross the placental barrier in some animal studies [11]. The safety of DEET in pregnancy is not established. There is evidence that it accumulates in fatty tissues and brain and there is a report of a child with mental retardation, impaired sensorimotor coordination and craniofacial dysmorphology born to a mother who had applied DEET daily throughout her pregnancy [12].

It is important to stress that malaria prophylaxis needs to be commenced 1 week before entry and continued for a further 4 weeks after leaving the malarial area. The combination recommended will depend on the area to be visited. In general, for low-risk areas such as North Africa, the Middle East and Central Asia, either a combination of proguanil and chloroquine or doxycycline is recommended. For variable-risk areas such as South and South East Asia, proguanil and chloroquine or mefloquine or Malarone (see below) are recommended. For high-risk areas such as Sub-Saharan Africa, mefloquine or Malarone are advised. However, not all of these are recommended for use in pregnancy (see Table 13.3).

Chloroquine (300 mg/wk) is regarded as safe in pregnancy, but single-agent therapy is becoming less effective. More areas of the world are becoming chloroquine resistant, and some areas multidrug resistant.

Pyrimethamine sulphadoxine marketed as Fansidar is no longer recommended because of its association with agranulocytosis,

Table 13.3 Malaria prophylaxis in pregnancy

Drug	Advise in pregnancy	Comments
Chloroquine	Safe in pregnancy	
Proguanil	Safe but recommend folate supplements	May be used in combination with chloroquine
Mefloquine	Avoid in first trimester	Reports of teratogenicity in animals studies
Malorpim (pyrimethamine and dapsone)	Not recommended in pregnancy	Possible teratogenic risk plus neonatal haemolysis
Doxycycline	Not recommended in pregnancy	
Malarone (proguanil and atovaquone)	Avoid unless essential	Limited information
Chinca alkaloids (quinine and quinidine	Not used for prophylaxis	Still have a place in the treatment of severe infections

and skin reactions including Stevens–Johnson syndrome and toxic epidermal necrolysis [13].

Mefloquine (250 mg/wk) should be avoided in the first trimester (or around the time of conception), as it has been shown to have teratogenic effects in animal studies. In trials using mefloquine later in pregnancy, there was a suggestion of an increase in the number of stillbirths, but this was not substantiated in further work [14,15].

Proguanil marketed as Paludrine (200 mg daily) would appear to be safe in pregnancy but is better used in combination therapy with chloroquine.

The newer drug *Malarone*, a combination of proguanil hydrochloride (100 mg) and atovaquone (250 mg) daily, has limited information with regard to pregnancy. It is not listed as contraindicated but best avoided unless essential [16].

The cinchona alkaloids *quinine* and *quinidine* have been associated with stillbirth and congenital abnormality and are therefore not recommended for use in pregnancy, although they still have a place in the treatment of severely infected pregnant women [17].

Similarly *doxycycline* is contraindicated particularly in the later stages of pregnancy as it affects skeletal development in animal studies and has clearly been shown to lead to dental discoloration in humans.

The areas which carry the highest risk of multidrug resistant malaria are East Africa, Thailand, Papua New Guinea and the Thai-Cambodia and Myanmar borders. Pockets of malaria are also found in Armenia, Azerbaijan, Georgia, Tajikistan and Turkmenistan. Women should be strongly advised against travelling to these areas during pregnancy.

Antibiotics and other anti-infective agents

Bacterial, viral, fungal and parasitic infections are not uncommon in pregnancy, with urinary tract infections being a particular risk, and drugs suitable for treatment of these conditions are discussed in Chapter 3. Antibiotics may be carried as part of a first-aid kit for travellers and in general the following may be considered for this purpose:

- Amoxycillin for urinary and upper respiratory infections.
- Metronidazole is a useful antiparasitic, particularly for the treatment of giardiasis and amoebiasis. Whilst it can be used for traveller's diarrhoea, it should probably not be carried in a first-aid kit to be administered without medical supervision. It should only be used when other therapeutic options are not available [18].
- The antifungal agents nystatin and Canestan can be safely used topically in pregnancy and should be part of the 'kit', particularly in hot climates where the incidence of vaginal candidiasis may be increased [19].

Table 13.4 gives and overview of the commonly used drugs for the treatment of traveller's diarrhoea and comments relating to their use in pregnancy [20].

Drugs that can be used for other common minor and self-limiting conditions are dealt with elsewhere in this publication and may be considered as part of the 'medical kit'.

Women taking other regular medications

In general, women taking other prescribed medications should be advised that all medications should be taken in their original containers and ensured that there are no restrictions on taking

Table 13.4 Drugs used for traveller's diarrhoea in pregnancy

Drug	Indication	Advice in pregnancy
Bismuth subsalycilate (Pepto-Bismuth)		Avoid
Loperamide (Imodium)	Watery diarrhoea	Safe
Diphenylate with atropine (Lomotil)	Watery diarrhoea	Use loperamide in preference
Piperazine (Antepar)	Antiparasitic	Contraindicated
Trimethoprim	Anti-infective (folate antagonist)	Case reports and controlled trails have not demonstrated increased fetal abnormality
Ciprofloxacin	Anti-infective	Safety not yet established
Metrinidazole	Giardiasis/amoebiasis	Use only if other therapeutic options not available
Quinacrine	Giardiasis	Contraindicated

them out of the country. Those women with pre-existing disease, hypertension, diabetes or renal conditions or who have a poor past obstetric history should be advised against long-distance travel, particularly to areas where medical attention may not be readily available.

All travellers should be advised to take with them a first-aid kit that should include a sterile medical pack containing sterile syringes and needles which can be bought over the counter at most good pharmacies. My suggestion for the contents of the first-aid kit are shown in Table 13.5.

Key points

- Immunisation should be given in pregnancy only if there is a clear indication and travel to an endemic area cannot be avoided
- No drug regimen ensures complete protection against malaria
- Women with pre-existing medical problems or a poor past obstetric history should be advised against long-distance travel

Table 13.5 Suggestions for the pregnant traveller's first-aid kit

Indication	Suggestion
General	Sterile medical pack
Travel sickness	Vitamin B6 or cyclizine
Malaria prophylaxis	Proguanil and chloroquine and folic acid
Diarrhoea	Loperamide (and metronidazole for use under medical supervision)
Thrush	Canestan pessary and cream
Urinary tract or upper respiratory tract infection	Amoxycillin
Analgesic	Paracetamol and codeine phosphate

References

1 Hurley P. Vaccination in pregnancy. *Curr Obstet Gynaecol* 1998;**8**:169–75.
2 Guidelines for vaccinating pregnant women. In: *Recommendations of the Advisory Committee on Immunization Practice (ACIP)*. Atlanta, GA: Center Disease Control & Prevention; 2002.
3 Immunological products and vaccines, Chapter 14. *British National Formulary, 51st edition*. London: Pharmaceutical Press; 2006:611–31.
4 Immunization in pregnancy. ACOG Committee Opinion No. 282. 2003.
5 Cholera. In: Salisbury D, Begg N (eds.), *Immunisation against Infectious Disease*. London: HMSO; 1996.
6 Tetanus. In: Salisbury D, Begg N (eds.), *Immunisation against Infectious Disease*. London: HMSO; 1996.
7 Samuel BU, Barry M. The pregnant traveller. *Infect Dis Clin N Am* 1998;**12**(2):325–54.
8 Watson JC, Fleming DW, Bordella AJ, et al. Vertical transmission of hepatitis A resulting in an outbreak in a neonatal intensive unit. *J Infect Dis* 1993;**167**(3):567–71.
9 Nelson-Piercy C. Chapter 11. In: *Handbook of Obstetric Medicine*. Oxford: Isis Medical Media; 1997:162.
10 Bloland PB, Wirima JT, Steketree RW, et al. Maternal HIV infection and infant mortality in Malawi: evidence for increased mortality due to placental malaria. *AIDS* 1995;**9**:721–6.
11 Blomquist L, Thorsell W. Distribution and fate of insect repellent 14C-*N,N*-diethyl-*m*-tolumide in the animal: II. Distribution and excretion after cutaneous application. *Acta Pharmacol Toxicol* 1977;**41**:235.
12 Sheafer C, Peters PW. Intrauterine diethyltoluamide exposure and fetal outcome. *Reprod Toxicol* 1992;**6**(20):175–6.
13 Clarification: Fansidar – not for malaria prophylaxis. *DTB* 1998;**36**:24.

14 Nosten F, ter Kuile F, Maelankiri L, et al. Mefloquine prophylaxis prevents malaria during pregnancy: a double-blind, placebo controlled-study. *J Infect Dis* 1994;**169**(3):595–603.
15 Phillips-Howard PA, Steffen R, Kerr L, et al. Safety of mefloquine and other antimalarial agents in the first trimester of pregnancy. *J Travel Med* 1998;**5**(3):121–6.
16 Radloff PD, Phillips J, Nkeyi M, et al. Atovaquone and proguanil for plasmodium faciparum malaria. *Lancet* 1996;**247**:1511.
17 McEvoy GK, Litvak K, Welsh OH, et al. (eds.). *American Hospital Formulary Service Drug Information*. Bethesda: American Society of Health – System Pharmacists; 1997.
18 Hammill HA. Metronidazole, clindamycin and quinolones. *Obstet Gynecol Clin North Am* 1989;**16**:531–40.
19 Rosa FW, Baum C, Shaw M. Pregnancy outcomes after first-trimester vaginitis drug therapy. *Obstet Gynecol* 1987;**69**(5):751–5.
20 Hurley PA. Travelling in pregnancy. *The Diplomate* 1999;**5**:254.

CHAPTER 14
Drugs in breastfeeding

Jane M. Rutherford

Drugs given to a breastfeeding mother may affect her baby. The drugs that have adverse effects on a breastfeeding infant may be different from those that cause problems in pregnancy since the mechanisms of transfer of compounds across the breast differ from those in the placenta. The most important factor is not necessarily whether the drug crosses into breast milk, but the concentration of drug in the blood of the infant and the effect that this might have.

As with the use of drugs during pregnancy, drug companies are generally unwilling to recommend the use of drugs during lactation because of problems with litigation and the ethical impossibility of performing randomised trials. Therefore, the information that is available about the effects on infants of drugs given to breastfeeding women is accumulated through case reports and series of varying size. Because of this, there is more information and experience regarding older drugs and relatively little about new compounds.

General principles

Maternal drug concentration

The obvious factors that affect maternal drug concentrations are drug dose, frequency, route of administration and patient compliance. Within 2 weeks of delivery, the majority of the physiological changes in the circulation that occur as part of pregnancy have reverted to the non-pregnant state. This means that in the first 2 weeks of lactation the plasma concentrations of drugs may vary considerably. Subsequent to this, plasma levels of water-soluble drugs will be similar to those in non-pregnant women. The changes

---

Prescribing in Pregnancy, 4th edition. Edited by Peter Rubin and Margaret Ramsay,
 ISBN: 978-1-4051-4712-5.

in body fat distribution take longer to revert to the pre-pregnant state. This results in the plasma concentrations of fat-soluble drugs tending to be lower during lactation than in the non-pregnant state.

Drug transfer across the breast

Most drugs will pass into breast milk in greater or lesser amounts. The amount of drug available for transfer across the breast will depend on blood flow to the breast. It is known that blood flow to the breast increases generally during lactation, but it is not clear whether there are variations in the blood flow during or between feeds [1]. Whether the drug molecules pass across the breast into the milk will then depend on the properties of the drug itself. Small molecules get into breast milk more easily than large ones. Fat-soluble, lipophilic drugs will pass across the cell membrane more easily than those with low lipid solubility. The degree of ionisation of the drug and the relative pH of maternal plasma and breast milk also play a role as does the relative affinity of the drug binding to milk and plasma proteins. In a few instances, active transport mechanisms across the breast have been detected [1]. In addition, there are some drugs that may be metabolised within the breast tissue and metabolites excreted into the milk [2].

Drug concentration in the infant

One of the factors determining how much drug a baby will ingest is the timing of feeds in relation to maternal dose schedule. The frequency, volume and duration of feeds are also important. The milk produced at the beginning of a feed (the foremilk) is protein rich and has a lower fat content to that at the end of a feed (the hindmilk). Therefore, there will be higher concentrations of fat-soluble drugs in the hindmilk. Babies who are fed longer will get increased amounts of such fat-soluble compounds compared to those who feed little and often [2]. Infant metabolism is immature compared to adults. Because of this, the half-life of some drugs in the neonatal circulation is longer than in the maternal blood. This may lead to accumulation of drug in the infant (see Figure 14.1).

Specific agents

The following lists and tables are by no means intended to be comprehensive, but I have included many of the commonly prescribed

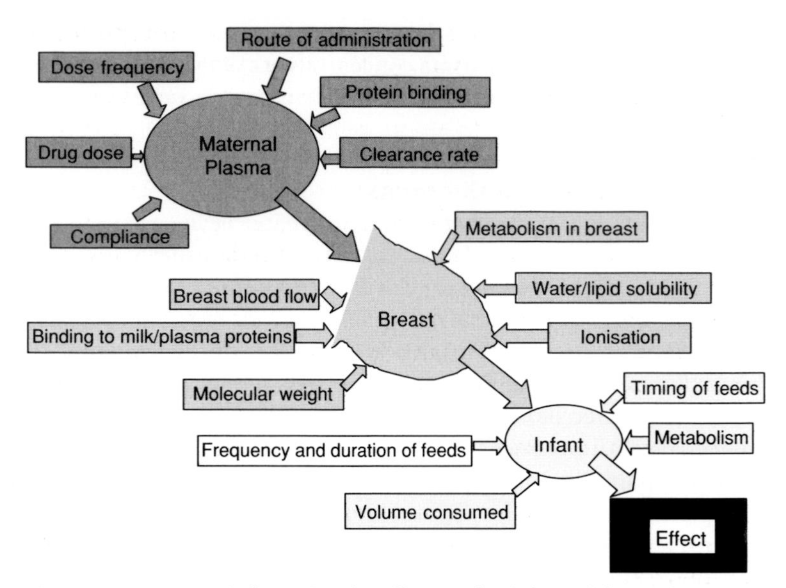

Figure 14.1 Factors influencing the effect on the infant of drugs given to the lactating mother.

drugs. In general, new drugs are to be avoided because of the likely lack of information regarding their safety. The information used in compiling these sections, except where specified, is gathered from references [1,3–9].

Antimicrobial agents

Any antimicrobial agent that is excreted into breast milk may cause an alteration in the infant's bowel flora and may thus cause diarrhoea. In addition, if the infant develops a pyrexia, it is important that maternal antimicrobial therapy is taken into account (see Table 14.1).

Analgesic drugs

Paracetamol is excreted into breast milk in very low concentrations, too small to have any effect on the infant and is therefore the safest analgesic available. *Aspirin* and salicylates are excreted into breast milk in low concentrations. However, because of immature metabolism, high concentrations could potentially accumulate in infant serum which may theoretically result in platelet dysfunction and Reye's syndrome. There is, however, only one report in the literature of salicylate toxicity in a breastfed infant despite extensive use. In view of the theoretical risks, analgesic doses of aspirin should probably be avoided since other agents are available. Where low-dose aspirin is used as thromboprophylaxis, then breastfeeding is probably safe.

There are no reports of adverse effects with the non-steroidal anti-inflammatory drugs *diclofenac, ibuprofen, mefenamic acid* and *naproxen* which are all excreted into breast milk in very low concentrations and are therefore safe during lactation. Although there was a single case of neonatal seizures in association with *indometacin* [10], no further such events have been identified. Only very small amounts are excreted into breast milk and it is therefore considered safe. Selective COX-2 inhibitors should be avoided as there are very few data available.

Opiates

Morphine is excreted into breast milk. It is unlikely to cause adverse effects in therapeutic doses. However, because of the immature infant metabolism, the half-life is prolonged and accumulation of the drug can occur. *Pethidine* and its active metabolite are excreted into breast milk. The half-lives are much longer in infants than in adults because of immature metabolism. Repeated doses, particularly in patient-controlled analgesia devices may lead to accumulation and cause neurobehavioural depression. Caution should therefore be exercised. *Fentanyl* and *alfentanyl* are safe to use in breastfeeding as the concentration in breast milk is negligible. *Codeine* passes into breast milk in concentrations which are of minimal significance, and it is therefore safe in breastfeeding (see Table 14.2).

Anticoagulant drugs

Heparin, because of its large molecular weight, is not excreted into breast milk. *Warfarin* is also not excreted into breast milk. Both of these agents are therefore safe for use in breastfeeding. There is little information on the effects of low-molecular-weight heparins on breastfed infants. However, there are unlikely to be any adverse effects since they have relatively high molecular weights and probably do not pass into breast milk. In addition, if they were present in the milk they would be inactivated in the infant's gastrointestinal tract. Other oral anticoagulants (for example, phenindione) should be avoided. For information on *aspirin*, see section on *Analgesic drugs*.

Table 14.1 Antimicrobials

Drug	Comments	Effect on infant	Safety in breastfeeding
Penicillin	Low concentrations in breast milk	No specific adverse effect	Safe
Cephalosporins	Low concentrations in breast milk	No specific adverse effect	Safe
Erythromycin	Excreted in breast milk	No specific adverse effect	Safe
Azithromycin	Excreted in a dose-dependent fashion	No adverse effects reported	Probably safe although little data
Tetracyclines	Low concentrations in breast milk	Theoretical risk of tooth discolouration and disruption of bone growth; unlikely in reality because of low infant serum concentration	Avoid if possible
Sulphonamides	Low concentrations in breast milk	Risk of kernicterus in preterm, ill or stressed infants	Safe in healthy term infants; avoid in preterm, ill or stressed neonates
Aminoglycosides	Present in breast milk and may be absorbed by infant in small amounts but absorption from gastrointestinal tract poor	No specific effect	Benefits probably outweigh risk
Metronidazole	Excreted into breast milk	Has been reported to give breast milk an unpleasant taste	Probably safe

Ciprofloxacin (and other quinolones)	Excreted into breast milk; oral doses concentrated in breast milk and produce milk levels higher than serum	Little good quality data but *Clostridium difficile* infection reported in a neonate of a mother taking ciprofloxacin; animal data suggest risk of arthropathy in infants	Avoid; allow 48 h after last dose before resuming feeding
Chloramphenicol	Excreted into breast milk	Potential risk of bone-marrow suppression; concentrations too low to cause the grey baby syndrome	Avoid
Acyclovir	Concentrated in breast milk; levels exceed those in maternal serum	No adverse effects identified	Probably safe, particularly as it is used to treat herpes virus infections in the neonate with no adverse effects
Antimalarial drugs	Excreted in low concentrations, not high enough to provide antimalarial protection to the infant	No adverse effects with the older drugs (*chloroquine*, *proguanil*); little data about *mefloquine*	*Chloroquine* and *proguanil* are considered safe; use *mefloquine* if benefits outweigh risks
Antituberculosis drugs	Excreted in low concentrations	No adverse effects with *ethambutol* and *rifampicin*; no data on *pyrazinamide*; theoretical risk of interference with nucleic acid function and hepatotoxicity with *isoniazid* but no adverse reactions reported	Probably safe

Table 14.2 Antihypertensives and other cardiovascular drugs

Drug	Comments	Effect on infant	Safety in breastfeeding
Hydralazine	Excreted into breast milk	No reported adverse effects	Considered safe
Nifedipine [11]	Low concentrations in breast milk	No reported adverse effects	Considered safe
Other calcium channel blockers	Little data	Little data	
Methyl dopa [12]	Excreted into breast milk in small amounts	No reported adverse effects	Considered safe
β-Blockers, propranolol, labetalol, metoprolol, atenolol	Excreted into breast milk; concentrated in breast milk [13,14]	No reports of adverse effects but theoretical risk of respiratory depression, bradycardia and hypoglycaemia; one report of features of β-blockade in infant where mother was taking atenolol [14]	β-Blockers are probably safe in conjunction with breastfeeding; infants should be observed for signs of β-blockade; it has been suggested that atenolol and metoprolol be avoided because of the high concentrations in milk [14,15]; however, there has been extensive use of atenolol with only one report of an adverse event and the risks are probably minimal

Thiazide diuretics	Low concentrations in breast milk	Large doses may suppress lactation	Safe in normal doses
Frusemide	Low concentrations in breast milk	No reports of adverse effects	Safe
Captopril, enalapril	Amounts in breast milk negligible	No reports of adverse effects	Probably safe
Other ACE inhibitors	Little data	Little data	
Angoitensin II receptor antagonists	No data	No data	Avoid because of lack of data
Amiodarone	Contains iodine; excreted into breast milk; long half-life in adults – unknown in neonates	Little data on infant effects but neonatal hypothyroidism has been reported	Avoid during breastfeeding; do not commence breastfeeding if the mother has taken amiodarone for prolonged periods within the preceding few months
Digoxin	Excreted into breast milk	No reports of adverse effects	Probably safe

Anti-asthmatic drugs

There are few data available on the effects of β-agonist drugs such as *salbutamol* and *terbutaline* particularly when taken by inhalation. However, no adverse reports have been located, and in view of the extent of the use of such drugs in women of childbearing age, it is likely that if adverse effects existed, they would have been detected. These drugs are therefore probably safe. For *salmeterol* there are also no data; however, it is unlikely that the neonate would ingest clinically significant amounts and it should therefore be considered safe.

Theophylline is excreted into breast milk in low concentrations. There is one report of irritability in an infant following ingestion of a rapidly absorbed aminophylline solution. Young infants may experience toxicity at lower levels than older infants. Slow-release preparations are therefore more likely to be well tolerated and caution should be exercised.

There are no reports of the effects of *inhaled steroids* on breastfed infants. However, since oral corticosteroids are considered safe, inhaled steroids are also probably safe.

Antihistamines

There are few reports on the effects of antihistamines on breastfed infants.

Anti-epileptic drugs

Phenytoin, carbamazepine and *sodium valproate* are excreted into breast milk. There is little risk to the neonate if drug levels in the mother are maintained within the therapeutic range. They are considered safe.

Phenobarbitone is excreted in breast milk, and because of immature infant metabolism, can accumulate in the infant. This can result in sedation. Withdrawal effects have also been observed after abrupt withdrawal of breastfeeding in a woman taking phenobarbitone. Breastfeeding should therefore be avoided if possible.

Lamotrigine is excreted into the breast milk. Some reports suggest that the concentrations of the drug in the infant are minimal [16]. However, others have found higher plasma concentrations in infants [17]. Lamotrigine is metabolised by glucuronidation which is immature in infants and therefore may result in significant accumulations [18] There are no reports of adverse effects in the infants of breastfed mothers taking lamotrigine; however, caution should be exercised because of the concerns from these studies.

There is no information about the effects of *gabapentin, vigabatrin* or *levetiracetam* in breastfeeding (see Table 14.3).

Gastrointestinal drugs

Drugs affecting gastric acid

Simple antacids are generally considered to be safe during breastfeeding. *Cimetidine* and *ranitidine* [19] are actively transported into breast milk with high milk-to-plasma ratios. However, the dose received by the infant is lower than that given to treat infant problems. There are no reports of adverse effects and they are therefore probably safe. *Omeprazole* enters human milk, but in low concentrations. There are no adequate reports regarding its effect on breastfeeding infants.

Laxatives

Laxative drugs that are absorbed from the maternal gastrointestinal tract may pass into the breast milk and cause diarrhoea in the infant. If laxatives are necessary, it is preferable to prescribe bulk laxatives such as ispaghula husk which are not absorbed.

Antiemetics

Prochlorperazine is probably secreted into breast milk. There are no data regarding adverse effects. There is also no information regarding *cyclizine*. However, since there are no reports of adverse effects with these drugs, and they have been available for a considerable time, they are probably safe. *Metoclopramide* is concentrated in breast milk. However, the total daily dose received by a breastfed infant of a mother receiving 30 mg/day is less than the dose recommended for therapeutic use in infants or premature neonates. The only adverse effects reported are two cases of mild abdominal discomfort. Although it is probably safe, caution should be exercised because of the theoretical central nervous system effects.

Drugs for inflammatory bowel disease

Mesalazine, suphasalazine and *olsalazine* are excreted in low concentrations into breast milk. Diarrhoea that resolved on stopping the drug has occurred in the infants of breastfeeding mothers taking these compounds. However, other adverse effects have not been

Table 14.3 Hormones and drugs used for endocrine conditions

Drug	Comments	Effect on infant	Safety in breastfeeding
Insulin	Does not pass into breast milk	None	Safe
Metformin	Low concentrations in breast milk	Unlikely to cause significant effects	Probably safe
Chlorpropamide/ tolbutamide	Excreted into breast milk	No reports of adverse effects but hypoglycaemia is a potential risk	Use only with caution
Thyroxine	Low concentrations in breast milk	Concentrations not high enough to protect the infant from neonatal hypothyroidism; may interfere with diagnosis of hypothyroidism on Guthrie test	Safe
Carbimazole/ methimazole	Excreted into breast milk	Theoretical risk of thyroid suppression; evidence suggests that if <15 mg/day is given to the mother then there is no effect on the infant	Lowest effective dose should be given; monitor infant thyroid function weekly
Propylthiouracil	Low concentrations in breast milk	No reports of adverse effects	Probably safe; monitor infant thyroid function
Radioactive iodine (I^{131})	Concentrated in breast milk	Can be taken up by infant thyroid and result in permanent thyroid damage	Contraindicated
Combined oral contraceptive pill	Oestrogen enters breast milk in concentrations less than physiological levels	No effect on infant but may shorten duration of lactation	Avoid because of effects on lactation
Progestogen only pill		No effect	Safe
Androgens/ antiandrogens	Pass into breast milk	May cause androgenic/antiandrogenic effects on infant	Contraindicated
Danazol		May cause androgenic effects on infant	Contraindicated

Table 14.4 Antipsychotic drugs, antidepressants and sedatives

Drug	Comments	Effect on infant	Safety in breastfeeding
Phenothiazines (chlorpromazine, flupenthixol, haloperidol)	Excreted into breast milk	Little data but may cause drowsiness and lethargy; theoretical effects of dopamine receptor antagonism on the developing central nervous system	No evidence to discontinue breastfeeding but caution should be exercised
Lithium	Excreted into breast milk in significant concentrations	No adverse effects reported but potential for toxicity is high; no studies of long-term effects	Use only with caution; controlling maternal drug levels will help to minimise risks; observe infant for signs of toxicity
Tricyclic antidepressants (amytriptyline, imipramine, desipramine)	Excreted into breast milk	Negligible concentrations detected in infant serum; no adverse effects reported	Probably safe but exercise some caution
Doxepin	Excreted into breast milk	Metabolites may accumulate in infant serum; one report of respiratory depression	Avoid if possible
Fluoxetine, sertraline, paroxetine, citalopram	Excreted into breast milk	Several studies have shown low serum concentrations in infants and no short-term developmental problems [21–24]; however, concerns exist about the long-term effects on neurobehaviour and development which are unknown	Probably safe, but exercise caution and monitor neonate for signs of adverse effects
Diazepam	Excreted into breast milk	May accumulate in the infant and lead to sedation; withdrawal may also cause adverse effects	Avoid
Temazepam	Excreted into breast milk	No adverse effects reported but risk of sedative effect if large doses given	Use only with caution; avoid breastfeeding if large amounts taken as drug of abuse

reported. These drugs are not contraindicated, but caution should be exercised when prescribing these drugs in breastfeeding and the infants should be observed carefully for changes in stool consistency.

Immunosuppressants

Prednisolone is excreted into the breast milk in small quantities [20]. It has been used extensively in breastfeeding women and there have been no reports of serious adverse effects. It is therefore considered safe.

Gold is excreted into breast milk and is absorbed by the infant. Adverse effects in infants such as rashes, nephritis, hepatitis and haematological abnormalities have been reported, but a causal relationship is not established. However, there is the potential for toxicity in the infant and caution should be exercised.

There are few data regarding other immunosuppressant drugs such as *azathioprine, methotrexate, cyclophosphamide* and *cyclosporin.* However, because of the high potential toxicity of these drugs, they should probably be avoided in breastfeeding, or lactation discontinued (see Table 14.4).

References

1 Wilson JT, Brown RD, Cherek DR, et al. Drug excretion in human breast milk: principles, pharmacokinetics and projected consequences. *Clin Pharmacokinet* 1980;**5**:1–66.

2 Wilson JT, Hinson JL, Brown D, Smith IJ. A comprehensive assessment of drugs and toxins in breast milk. In: Hamosh M, Goldman AS (eds.), *Human Lactation 2: Maternal and Environmental Factors*. New York: Plenum Press; 1986.

3 Bennet PN, the WHO Working Group. *Drugs and Human Lactation: A Guide to the Content and Consequences of Drugs, Micronutrients, Radiopharmaceuticals and Environmental and Occupational Chemicals in Human Milk.* Amsterdam: Elsevier Science; 1988.

4 Briggs GG, Freeman RK, Yaffe SJ. *Drugs in Pregnancy and Lactation.* Baltimore: Williams and Wilkins; 1998.

5 Committee on Drugs. The transfer of drugs and other chemicals into human milk. *Pediatrics* 1994;**93**:137–50.

6 Lee JJ, Rubin AP. Breast feeding and anaesthesia. *Anaesthesia* 1993;**48**:616–25.

7 Pons G, Rey E, Matheson I. Excretion of psychoactive drugs into breast milk. *Clin Pharmacokinet* 1994;**27**:270–89.

8 Smith IJ, Wilson JT. Infant effects of drugs excreted into breast milk. *Pediatr Rev Commun* 1989;**3**:93–113.

9 Weiner CP, Buhimschi C. *Drugs for Pregnant and Lactating Women*. Philadelphia, PA: Churchill Livingstone; 2004.

10 Eeg-Olofsson O, Malmros I, Elwin CE, Steen B. Convulsions in a breast-fed infant after maternal indomethacin. *Lancet* 1978;**2**:215.

11 Ehrenkranz RA, Ackerman BA, Hulse JD. Nifedipine transfer into human milk. *J Pediatr* 1989;**114**:478–80.

12 White WB, Andreoli JW, Cohn RD. Alpha-methyl dopa disposition in mothers with hypertension and in their breast fed infants. *Clin Pharmacol Ther* 1985;**37**;387–90.

13 Liedholm H, Melander A, Bitzen P-O, et al. Accumulation of atenolol and metoprolol in human breast milk. *Eur J Clin Pharmacol* 1981;**20**:229–31.

14 Schmimmel MS, Eidelman AJ, Wilschanski MA, Shaw D, Ogilvie RJ, Koren G. Toxic effects of atenolol consumed during breast feeding. *J Pediatr* 1989;**114**:476–8.

15 Anderson PO. Letter. *Pediatrics* 1995;**95**:957.

16 Rambeck B, Kurleman G, Stodieck SRG, May TW, Jurgens U. Concentrations of lamotrigine in a mother on lamotrigine treatment and her newborn child. *Eur J Clin Pharmacol* 1997;**51**;481–4.

17 Tomson T, Ohman S, Vitols S. Lamotrigine in pregnancy and breastfeeding. *Epilepsia* 1997;**38**;1039–41.

18 Liporace J, Kao A, D'Abreu A. Concerns regarding lamotrigine and breastfeeding. *Epilepsy Behav* 2004;**5**:102–5.

19 Oo CY, Kuhn RJ, Desai N, McNamara PJ. Active transport of cimetidine into human milk. *Clin Pharmacol Ther* 1995;**58**;548–55.

20 Ost L, Wettrall G, Bjorkhelm I, Rane A. Prednisone excretion in human milk. *J Pediatr* 1985;**106**:1008–11.

21 Yoshida K, Smith B, Craggs M, Kumar RC. Fluoxetine in breast milk and developmental outcome of breastfed infants. *Br J Psychiatry* 1998;**172**:175–8.

22 Heikkinen T, Ekblad U, Palo P, Laine K. Pharmacokinetics of fluoxetine and norfluoxetine in pregnancy and lactation. *Clin Pharmacol Ther* 2003;**73**:330–7.

23 Stowe ZN, Cohen LS, Hostetter A, Ritchie JC, Owens MJ, Nemeroff CB. Paroxetine in human breast milk and nursing infants. *Am J Psychiatry* 2001;**158**:144–5.

24 Berle JO, Steen VM, Aamo TO, Breilid H, Zahlsen K, Spigset O. Breastfeeding during maternal antidepressant treatment with serotonin reuptake inhibitors: infant exposure, clinical symptoms and cytochrome P450 genotypes. *J Clin Psychiatry* 2004;**65**;1228–34.

Index